NEUROPHILOSOPHY OF CONSCIOUSNESS, VOL. VI

THE EVOLUTION OF COMPLEXITY IN 4-D SPACE TIME

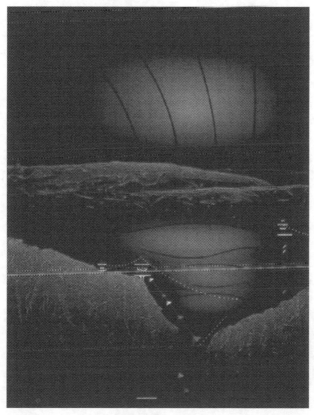

The Biosphere

Dr. Angell de la Sierra, Esq.

Order this book online at www.trafford.com
or email orders@trafford.com

Most Trafford titles are also available at major online book retailers.

Printed in the United States of America.

ISBN: 978-1-4669-9342-6 (sc)
ISBN: 978-1-4669-9341-9 (e)

Trafford rev. 05/16/2013

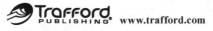

www.trafford.com

North America & international
toll-free: 1 888 232 4444 (USA & Canada)
phone: 250 383 6864 ♦ fax: 812 355 4082

CONTENTS

Ramblings on a Reality Check

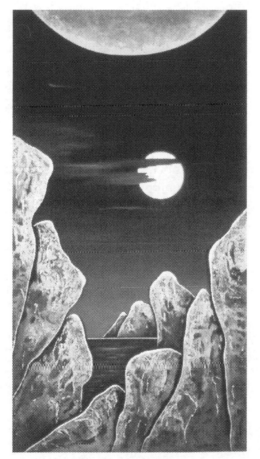

Lunar Landscape

PROLOGUE

This brief prologue represents the bridging link from the epilogue of previous Vol. V (Part I) of this series and the current Vol. VI as we continue to disentangle the complexities of the human mind-brain dynamics as it adjusts/equilibrates—in the biopsychosocial (BPS) realm—to a continuously evolving existential reality. As we witness the increasing polarization between the pragmatic phenomenological realism of the health/engineers/legal professional practitioners and the idealized epistemological conjectures/speculations of the equivalent arm chair theorists, we further realize why the human species, not withstanding its relatively inferior biological survival potential when compared to other advanced subhuman species, has managed to carry on the baton of evolutionary progress in medicine, engineering and law throughout recorded history. How else can anyone explain this apparent paradox other than by experiencing the successful collective efforts of the 'hands on practitioners' and the 'arm chair theorists'. Why should an immediate ontological, materialistic physics exclude a transcendental metaphysics logic . . . or vice verse? Why not settle for a hybrid Epistemontological ecumenism dealing with both the 'the seen **and** the unseen'? Unless, of course, the reader is acting 'politically' to advance his own selfish interests and thus ignoring Will Durant "Lessons of History." admonition about its consequences of having to repeat same errors. But, again, maybe the reader doesn't care about the future of the unborn of future generations and leave the future to better adapted subhuman species, e.g., ants, roaches, etc. who'd rather eat, stay alive, cavort in happy delight and become socially accepted in your pack. A veritable godless biopsychosocial (BPS) paradise! But, some of us believe there will be a brighter tomorrow lead by consciously good-willed individuals who feel responsible for their own just code of ethics and morality. It is not in the solitude of the laboratory practice that we learn to empathize, understand, tolerate and forgive. Likewise, it is not always possible that a human being is capable of overcoming the inherited limiting circumstances of the genetic endowment or controlling the acquired abnormal circumstances of his internal body-proper and/or the external environmental circumstances s(he) found when born. This ego driven underlying circumstantial background is what inspires 'the survival of the fittest' strategy for the 'political' extremists in our midst. Interestingly, Part II of previous Vol. V, (Yogi) fictionalizes how it may be possible to survive and sublimate deep pain and frustration into creative work. Enjoy.

"This Volume V (Neurophilosophy of Consciousness) is a continuation of the previous published volume that did not make it into press on time and represents an update on the status of consciousness as viewed within the context of an evolving perspective of human brain dynamics as evidenced by both modern technologies and new mathematical abstractions. One thing has been clear to this author, yes this is a 'Brave New World' worth discovering but we are shifting our emphasis too much into the vagaries of metaphysical abstractions at the expense of losing the ontological perspective of that evolving brain dynamics that makes it possible. It would seem as if our new physical materialist theoretical physicists and philosophers prefer to ignore that historical revolution that put man and his ongoing existential circumstances back at the center of the universe, like Husserl's phenomenology, e.g., Heidegger's existentiale Analytik, Ortega y Gasset's 'perspectivism', Dilthey's Leben philosophie and others. It is like ignoring that it was a human brain existing in a continuously evolving dynamic process of self transformation continues to un-relentlessly modify and reformulate his understanding of life experiences, rejecting the notion that if it was valid for the preceding 'classic' generation it is still viable in the modern convulsive 21th.century today.

The work of these 'existentialists' was mostly based on the lessons learned from recorded history but, important as it is as a source, we have to remember that history is a synthesis of facts where psychosocial circumstances heavily influenced human motives, behaviors and retaliations, i.e., historical facts are not necessarily objectively based on falsifiable facts in evidence. Likewise, the laws of nature are not necessarily always determined by the same particles interacting under similar circumstances. These two extreme positions need a contemporaneous update before they are reconciled and ultimately hybridized into a coherent Epistemontological unit whole. Neither should we accept the supremacy of the general, abstracts conceptualizations endorsed by materialist physics nor its total rejection as 'irrelevant' by radical empiricists that rather opt for the Sartrean type of day in and day out hedonistic existentialism. The temporality of evolutionary phenomenological and metaphysical logic change is very much part of reality. Natural events seem to repeat in cycles but only in appearance because the complete cycle was more of a spiral than a circle of repetition. As discussed *below in the Einstein-Bohr debate on the reality of the simultaneous verification of a particle's position and momentum, the verifiable 'here and now' is as important as the hypothesized predictable 'later', one reality but at different times, the verifiable present is best understood than an unverifiable conceptualization, albeit predictable (always?). In our BPS model we welcome the verifiable measurement or observation along with the transcendental reduction (Husserl's abstract analogical transposition) as the best compromise for a fundamental basis in the understanding the experience of reality

The logic behind this Epistemontological approach is simple, the human existential reality experienced is an individualized elaboration of the brain as determined by genetic, learned and yet undefined other possible influences that theosophical credo thrive on in their modeling of biopsychosocial poems, ergo human life is the ultimate reality. Consequently, the biopsychosocial equilibrium with circumstantial conditions that we share with the living subhuman species is necessary for day to day survival but not sufficient to guarantee the human species survival across generations. Unfortunately that guarantee is predicated on an efficient functional formulation of that relevant, falsifiable reality outside perceptual and/or conceptual threshold. It is not enough to exclusively study the details of human biopsycho social equilibrium (Ortega's metaphysics of the 'elan vital'), but neither is the exclusive abstract reduction to symbolic formulation of invisibilities, relevant or not, like extreme radical religionists do, theosophies and materialist physicists alike. Humans need not become the willing prisoners of the theoretical physicists' objectivism nor the biological research scientist objectivism to feed the ego of their intellectual proponents because existence is inexorably about both real perspectives, no principle can be superior to life . . . , all lives. To quote Ortega y Gasset: ". . . . , "my life"—in the "biographical" not in the "biological" sense—is the question of what to do with it and that of what happens to me as I find myself "shipwrecked" in the precarious sea of "circumstances."

For unknown reasons beyond my capacities to analyze, our human species has been uniquely endowed with the means to survive thanks to his introspective ability to ". . . sink into the inner depths of his being as he or she makes an effort to hold on to consciousness and to the very essence of his life . . . . (because) "To live," . . . "is to deal with the world, aim at it, act in it, be occupied with" (Obras, 5: 26, 33-34, 35, 44-45, 7: 103-04, Ortega). As we argue, the experience of existential living is not about some scientific description of fMRI brain recordings or some metaphysical logic principle underlying such observations unless the real life historical and psychosocial dimensions are incorporated into the equation.

For those respectful colleagues of mine in academia who keep insisting that my strategy all along—based on my publications—has consisted on deliberately or subconsciously marketing a Roman Catholic cosmogony without calling it by name, I rest on the literal interpretation of my writings by others in the general public. Like everyone else, we all have preferences that may be relevant or not to a particular domain of discourse. If nothing else it proves my point about judgments based on other than factual data as briefly mentioned below in relation to quantum non-locality. We all have beliefs that are based on individualized circumstances surrounding our cultural upbringing and adult life. That diagnosis on my 'hidden agenda' certainly is not based on signs and symptoms consistently observed or measured because one can be objective in recognizing meaningful content in those opposed to one's views. There existed many good human beings much before organized religions were established.

In any event we hope to have confused readers as much as we still remain ourselves about what the universal guiding principle should be as circumstances evolve into the future. What is or should be the ultimate criterion of truth for the faithful in the JudeoChrIslamic or physical materialist religions? We can also respect the Buddhist conviction that ultimately reality transcends all possible human elaborations and cannot ever be fully comprehended by sensory descriptions or linguistic and conceptual explanation, i.e., it escapes the grasp of language and thoughts representations for analysis. However, while we recognize the human brain sensory and conceptual limitations, it seems unwarranted to conclude that physical objects do not phenomenologically exist or emerge from non-physical empty vacuums.

Another issue worthwhile pointing out and discussed is this dilemma of 'which reality is true', if either one. The answer is related to the required reconciliation between quantum theory and general relativity. As we interpret it, the 'criterion of reality' seems to be related to the EPR and Bell's theorem interpretations (based on Bohm's spin measurements) of the physical real-time immanent 'locality' (as measured in the lab) and the hoped-for metaphysical universality of an alleged 'non-locality', the classical syndrome of confusing the reality of the conceptually inferred map with the reality of the phenomenologically perceptual territory. If we could only simultaneously measure or at least predict both the evolving and interacting variables then they can be regarded as simultaneous elements of physical reality, seen or unseen. But this is not yet the case for our limited human brain performance, which reality is true?

For the benefit of those more familiar with theoretical physics, the Einstein-Podolsky-Rosen 'solution' constituted an attempt of reconciliation of the phenomenological with the metaphysical has itself added new layers of confusion when attempting to solve the dilemma between a particle locality and quantum theoretical completeness by affirming the physical existence of a reality assumed (momentum) based on measurements of other presumably linked and interacting particle position. Needless to say that Einstein's strategy of maintaining locality is more appealing phenomenologically. On the other hand it would appear, from the Bell theorem adoption of Bohm's measurements on spin pairing suggesting non-locality, that Einstein's immanent sensory reality of experiencing locality consciously coexist with the mathematical logic of Bell's inequalities and the 'simultaneous' technological measuremens of observers miles apart! What description/explanation is incomplete? Which reality is true, Einstein's 'separability and local' appealing to phenomenological reality or the 'functionally linked and non-local' counterpart? Is it possible to modify the wave function such that mesoscopic reality becomes a hybrid incorporating both the phenomenological physical locality and the metaphysical non-locality? Stay tuned! End of Ch. 1

Immanent and Transcendental Issues in a Socio-political Philosophy

A Call for a Real-time Evolving Compromise

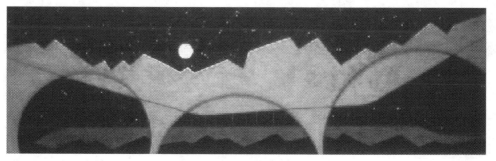

The Bridge

INTRODUCTION

Never before did the American voter have to choose between two extreme idealistic political philosophies as consistently evident from opinion polls when viewed by the average middle class moderate as a standard guide for a healthy, happy and convivial life for all NOW. For the first time most voters think both candidates are likeable family guys with what seems to half of the voters as a clear agenda to solve the immediate problems of the nation. If elected, will either one succeed in carrying on their policies on a both a current and a long range basis? We think not for the reasons explained below, unless they veer from their stated course and seriously consider the incorporation of the opposing candidate's logical viewpoints. To have the best of both approaches succeed we need to eventually let the loser of the election become automatically the vice-president and let the nation benefit from the presence of hybrid ideologies complementing each other as they coexist and evolve with unavoidable circumstances. Presidential candidates need to stop fighting the quixotic windmills of the opposing views as if they were necessarily relevant evils. I hope to provide below not an instant simplistic solution but an analytical insight as to what influential elements are the result of each candidate's inherited and environmentally acquired data base inputs into their decision-making process plus other relevant considerations as how to escape the subhuman manifold into eventual greater biopsychosocial (BPS) horizons for the human species.

ARGUMENTATION

It is naturally expected by the voters that once the national challenges to be encountered are spelled out and compared with the applicable philosophical model, the result will provide a moderate landscape for all appropriate adjustments to social contingencies predicted or considered as they arise; the same priority-based guidance both leader-protagonists would execute themselves in response to identical circumstances. As individuals, their intellectual fitness to the socio-political challenges ahead is of the essence and it depends on the genetic and acquired baggage they bring on to bear on the specific circumstantial challenges confronted and how they may logically transcend their BPS default responses in benefit of those they aspire to serve. Now get ready for the flight of fancy to follow.

Two individuals may have equivalent levels of fitness even when having very different sets of physical characteristics because intellectual fitness for a leadership job is an irreducible primitive trait that derives its meaning from the quasi axiomatic formulation of current/ ongoing socio-economic evolution theory that both candidates should have adopted in principle regardless of trivial priorities in their possible execution. Both candidates together and with the assistance of experts in economy and philosophy should be committed to distinguish the conflicting strands in the debate and minimize the unnecessary confusion that controls the media on the methodological role of economic optimality assumptions, and the explanatory goals of socioeconomic theory.

Besides, it has to be understood that individual hopefuls are not to be taken necessarily as instances of the general conceptualized human species anymore than Charlie Boy, my dog, should be taken as an instance of the generalized dog species. Every human being always carries with him/her the circumstances of their individualized biopsychosociology wherever s(he) goes and it would be misleading to assume that such individualized recipe will necessarily control their decision-making process. But, we need not a new set of natural laws for each individualized member of the human species. We need instead a compromise between the immanent satisfaction of real-time exigent circumstances and the assurance that such is consistent with the transcendental viability of the human species. Oil and vinegar won't mix unless you keep shaking the mixture or adding a common element with both hydrophobic and hydrophilic features and then crossing your fingers. For starters, the expert advisers need to identify which essential and specific exemplar mechanisms in one model are equivalent, not necessarily identical, to mechanisms in the other model adopting the same, or equivalent interphases representing the fundamental units of consensus and compromise whose usefulness may conceivably extend into a wide range of multidisciplinary solutions.

Now that I have outlined the predominantly biological imperatives that control the subhuman aspects of our existential reality I am moving into more complex psychosocial variables.

Anyone that has analytically observed the social behavior of any subhuman species must have noticed the human equivalent of 'nationality' in the territorial 'behavior' and the human equivalent of racial discrimination when a given species keeps away any other differently looking intruders into their turf which they will defend like modern terrorists do. Contrary to the popular classical interpretations to the effect that racial discrimination is exclusively learned, I dare say that the inherited and acquired aspects of BPS survival of the good but uneducated or unemployed hungry are manipulated by the special interests, whether political or economic which in the USA unfortunately identify the elected politicians which seem as if they surrender (for sale) before the clever manipulations by the special monopolistic capitalism economic interests that seems to control the elected government. The only way to escape that unintentional subhuman trap often imposed on the needy is the early indoctrination in ethics and morality by parents and organized religions for the benefit of those blessed with the natural talent to transcend the immanent biological imperative and become responsible leaders in their chosen disciplines. Who is at fault, the responsible self conscious business entrepeneur and libertarian idealist or the socialist leaning idealist? Neither one, even dogs and cats can learn to live together in the feral relationship of a healthy, happy and convivial compromise. It is a falsifiable fact, the rule we humans can make it to work just by trying. For those few prophets that recorded history has given that role, it seems like natural intelligence is necessary but not sufficient. Do we need the mediation of now unknown transfinite sources of righteousness inspiration to mediate in behalf of human survival as a viable species? Quare. The last two centuries have witnessed unsuspected 'miracles' in science and technology, and the show goes on with the help of quantum theory, metaphysical logic and an undefined mechanism of reciprocal information transfer between our prefrontal cortex space phase and transfinity as outlined elsewhere by the undersigned.

Continuing with the justification for a hybrid model approach to reconcile two worthwhile idealistic models of effective biopsychosocial (BPS) survival of the human species we now try to understand better why we all need to appreciate why there is an ethical and moral obligation beyond self gratification even though we recognize the subconscious pressures for a BPS equilibrium survival within the current and ongoing existential reality. We need to briefly examine the meaning of liberty for the two extreme functional ideologies. A dispassionate analysis will show that both extremes can properly claim the convenience of been guaranteed an unrestricted freedom from unjustified obstacles, barriers or constraints on free speech and peaceful demonstrations in act or potency. After all it should be the aim of all normal and consciously responsible citizens to invoke free will and take control of their lives and realize its fundamental BPS purposes. To negate these fundamental freedoms to others is symptomatic and/or diagnostic of the pursuit of unearned conveniences at the expense of innocent others. We see these behaviors more often associated with abusive individual agents or their collectivities, at both extremes of the ideological spectrum. These extremes are both the expression of a free conscious ideal about political liberty and autonomy, however incompatible the respective interpretations may be but they both necessarily agree on the pursuit of liberty for the individual to realize his highest aspirations individually or with the intervention of the state machinery. Can these two conflicting concepts of liberty be reconciled? Once we identify their common denominator what remains is to catalogue their differences as fundamentally essential or operational conveniences. Having identified their common lofty goal to pursue, how do they get there? Is getting there a mere possible or probable outcome? Obviously it depends on the individual and his real time circumstances to effectively deal with the anticipated or new constraints and the assigned priority, all things considered, to realize that goal. One can for instance rely on realizing one's true self, health or diseased, inside an underdeveloped socioeconomic environment or taking advantage of more sophisticated resources to plan your honest or corrupt strategies based on existing rational and well informed data bases. The big problem is not to realize that both conditions coexist in the same nation and consequently it is futile to use same remedy for different diseases when present. It is like importing a constitutional form of government and parliamentary elections after a constitutional assembly referendum among the Australian aborigenes! For those that argue that self realization attitudes, not environmental constraints is the determining factor are denying the fundamental plurality and diversity of the USA and consequently equating push genes with racial superiority. But, as sociology statistics records reveal, the shy impoverished citizen in backward communities becomes the entrepeneurial leader of the next generation given the opportunities and help from tax funded governmental programs. The beliefs, desires and values as taught at home, organized community and religious groups, government endorsed or not, and all together will play a major role in strengthening the shared commonalities. It is this real time diversity that negates the exclusivity of the free individual that takes the initiative to develop and take control of his essential needs and convenient desires and interests autonomously and from within. What about those who, through no conscious choice of their own, cannot enjoy that status as 'free individuals' that triggers autonomy and self realization? Should they continue in their perpetual role as in Alexander Dumas 'Les Miserables', or Raspails "The Condemned of the Earth." For those who, through no conscious effort of their own, inherited their socioeconomic status as 'free individuals', their lasting entrepeneurial success depends on reaching out to the 'miserables' not only as paternalistic and/or authoritative potential consumers of their products but as potential future happy partners in business. Instead, business leaders should join elected government in providing workfare opportunities, not welfare handouts. It is very difficult to formulate decisions on the basis of calm rational reflection on all the options available in the presence of socioeconomic pressures, manipulations by the combined forces of politicians and special interests or outright ignorance. Why insist by indoctrination or clever manipulation, e.g., arbitrary taxation, that there is only one American socioeconomic, sociopolitical and religious way of life instead of providing outlets for healthy, civil and moral expressions that do not compromise the basic values of ethical and moral conviviality and thereby taking into consideration the individualized needs and content of his cultural desires, whatever they are? Denying these outlets of expression negates constitutional freedom. In a free pluralistic society the national interests need not necessarily equate the individualized interests of its members in all respects and with the passage of time evolutionary pressures will control the direction of peaceful change and bring more creative uniformity, if any, by free choice or peaceful consensus. Just like there exist ecumenical theosophical convivialities, why shouldn't there be the sociopolitical equivalent? One could even conceive the extreme situation where an ecumenical partnership between free enterprise and a government of different political ideologies as suggested here could even impose specific and relevant dictatorial restraints to effectively deal with a temporary emergency without exercising arbitrary restraints on the liberty of the majority with impunity. There are historical records of these creative experiments of peaceful coexistence during the interface of an evolved and mature ancient Roman Empire and the surge of Renaissance forces of renewal and change. This should not be construed as an endorsement of one party society. Basic political differences should always have their separate for a of expression as we now have with independent Republican and Democrat parties each ideally committed to freedom and liberal democratic institutions free from the self-serving influence of powerful private enterprises of monopolistic capitalism waving their international green dollar flag of a global imperialistic economy state where its members have no country allegiances. We are suggesting this hybrid model on the premise that there should not be a fundamental difference between the Republican and the Democrat conceptualization of essential freedoms. The alternatives to peaceful ecumenical and political coexistence are clear and well documented by the Middle East tribal wars in Syria, Iraq, Afghanistan, Pakistan and the brewing expectations of economic instability of the Euro currency as triggered in no small context by the massive infiltration of 'non-documented illegal aliens' in Central Europe.

SUMMARY AND CONCLUSIONS

The Constitutional guarantees of individualized freedom to all members of a pluralistic society like ours should be the goal of any elected ideology. When different socio-economic ideologies can constructively and creatively interact it guarantees that all people enjoy minimal equal freedoms. By stimulating pre-election debates on socioeconomic models to solve the problems of all citizens in either side of the political debate and assuring that the presidential loser will become the automatic vice-president. It guarantees a healthy consideration of strategies to attend the basic needs of all represented as a function of available resources and established priorities.

REFERENCES

1. Erich Fromm. Man for Himself. 1947 Fawcett Premier Book.
2. Anthony Storr Human Aggression 1970 Bantam Books
3. John Oesterle Ethics. The Introduction to Moral Science. 1957 Prentice Hall
4. John L ocke Essays on Civil Government (Spanish) 1969 Aguilar
5. Dr. Angell de la Sierra Cabeza de Cordero o Rabo de Leon 2000 (Novel) Lulu
6. ". . . de la Libertad y Otras Ilusiones (Novel) Lulu

Dr. Angell O. de la Sierra, Esq. Deltona, Florida Summer, 2012-09-16

End of Ch. 2

My Credo, a Reply to a Learned Critique

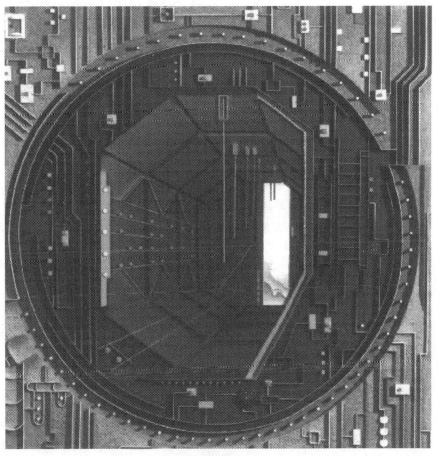

Virtual Reality

Prof. Chris King: "Angell . . . . , Aren't we all safer being part of a robust cosmological life process in which life has a central cosmological role of becoming? . . . ."

Angell: Wow! I have to share your insights with my family and friends Chris. Thanks a lot for taking all this time to read and reflect on my 'transcendental reciprocal information transfer between transfinity and human neocortex' sub model on life and consciousness.

Here's a brief reply for now. It was very impressive and I dare say it is difficult to disagree with most of your analysis. Your quote above has been for me a lifetime source of curiosity and driving force to search for credible answers satisfying both theists and atheists appetite, for IMHO, we are all believers in representing and structuring/modeling the relevant super-complex but invisible forces (beyond sensory perception or brain combinatorial resolution) influencing our quotidian existential reality. This because we, like all biota, are unconsciously (genetically) driven to preserve the integrity and viability of a reproductive biological life and subconsciously (memetically) driven to attain a psychic well being state and thereby emerge as a convivial and socially acceptable member of our 'tribes'. Three published volumes on "Neurophilosophy of Consciousness, a BPS Brain Dynamics Model." details it. Unlike these animals, the human species 'evolved', in addition, the capacity for an introspective search of self, aka self-consciousness', thanks to the co-evolution of the language machinery. This marvelous capacity to simultaneously become actor and critical observer of our willed, chosen adaptive responses to challenges to our biopsychosocial equilibrium in the environment, is strictly a human species gift. Unlike other species, it gives humans the unique capacity to transcend the biological enslavement of a reflex-driven existence, so aptly described by conditional learned responses models (Skinner, etc.). What will never fit this reflex-conditioned controlled life is the historically recorded events of humans as transcending the chains of self-serving biopsychosocial conveniences and engaging in self-conscious acts of altruism against such reflex driven acts protecting species survival self interests. You have heard and read this 'babble' before from me but consider that it is in harmony with your opening quote above. You would agree that ontological measurements from falsifiable observations are more reliable than mystical conjectures or speculations. But, how do we deal with the relevant but invisible forces in our midst that daily influence our existential reality? I suggest instead, in addition to the scientific methodology, metaphysical logic representations and elaborations (permutations, combinations, etc.), an epistemological approach to assist in dealing with that important self-evident invisibility influencing our lives that we experience but escapes our sensory or instrumental detection and description. Consequently, human realism is a hybrid Epistemontological experience we can use, especially at the mesoscopic level to improve on the quality of real-time living.

However, the highly successful quantum theoretical 'scientific methodology', is responsible for many useful developments and it all started (and continues!) with abstract representations of the invisible but extrasensory experienced falsifiable probabilistic event. How is, e.g., an invisible and alleged adimensional point singularity or its spatial Planck-size extension string, vibrating at different frequencies, different from a dark baryonic DNA/RNA (variously explained as remnants of post Big Bang nucleo-synthetic activity, etc.)?. Assuming this brain fart is probable, I was asking for your mathematical insight to criticize, not the assumption, but the magnetic/electric conductance/flux roadways to handle the reciprocal information transfer. But you and Dr. RR Yanniru lightly dismissed the possibility of the assumption and period! Then I pressured you into expanding on my real Christian motivations, even when I never talked about religion. I was only indirectly pressing the materialist physicalists to be consistent, either they admit 1. causal connections between sequentially connected events, e.g., inorganic matter→living biota and 2. sequences progressing in the direction of ordered complexity cannot be spontaneously originated and sustained. Rational logic and a good familiarity with natural laws argues in favor of a causal driving force defying the entropy laws of nature. If in addition you experience happiness when you believe in loving your mother, God, your children, wife, dog, neighbor, etc. then you are doubly blessed!!! But if an atheist believes otherwise and truly feels happy about it, he is also a believer and may God(s) bless him too! Amen, Angell

Family Domain site: http://delaSierra-Sheffer.net

Blog site: http://angelldls.wordpress.com/

Prof. Chris King:

"Angell, To give you and the others on this list your true money's worth of insight in difficult times, let me give you a revolutionary take on the transcendental cosmology of God, life the universe and everything.

A couple of days ago, for the first time for a couple of years (because I myself am also frightened of my mind being torn apart by transcendence), I took the very best of sacred mushrooms and they gave me yet again a complete vision of how cosmic consciousness is coming about in the universe in one of the cleanest and strongest experiences I have ever had.

I won't go into all the incidental details of the retinal circus, including being transported to join God in heaven, with Saint Peter on a stage ushering me into the sanctum on a kind of dance stage a little like a new Orleans jazz routine, but the overwhelming power, detailed truth and integrity of the experience convinced me, yet again, firstly that the living sacraments contain the genuine royal blood route to religious knowing, and secondly that I have a personal responsibility to turn the tables on the false and fraudulent traditions of the pagan divine Lord that dominate Western Christian culture for the sake of life itself.

Now let's get to the details. How it works is this. The universe is a complementarity, in which subjective consciousness and the objective universe complement one another. Without this cosmic complementarity, our personal experience has no meaning, or real existence. It is also what the Upanishads and virtually all Eastern teachings say.

Now the interesting turning inside out bit is this. To fulfill conscious realization requires a complex inversion of physical cosmology, beginning with the mandala of the symmetry-broken forces of nature, leading to a fractal quantum architecture of atoms, molecules, biogenesis and ultimately tissues and organisms through the evolutionary process.

Only then can cosmogenesis begin to manifest subjective consciousness through the sappy holographic biochemical brain, which has evolved to make animals able to anticipate future threats to survival in the computationally intractable open environment through processes which most plausibly are happening through space-time entanglement at the quantum level thus manifesting the cosmic complementarity that set this whole thing off. There is no way this can be reduced to a purely electrochemical phenomenon or a bit based computation like a von Neumann computer.

Now, in this process, cosmic consciousness can and does arise only through the individual subjective consciousness of the biota. There is no independent third party personality of God pulling the marionette strings, but there is a natural propensity in human consciousness for religious experience, because, although the brain has to close down the doors of perception sufficiently to enable subjective consciousness to protect organismic survival, it can't do it completely, because the brain evolved so the doors of perception were open enough to anticipate reality.

Consequently people throughout history have had a gathering sense that there is a transcendental conscious reality burgeoning up within their individual consciousness and try to talk about it in terms of deities, God, supernatural spirits and psychic influences, thus giving rise to the major world religions and to the false deification of Jesus as transcendental messiah in the pagan Hellenistic tradition of Paul.

The end result is that God exists only in so far as we can enter into deeper more cosmic forms of subjective consciousness in which the egotistical bundle of life becomes loosened enough so that our personal consciousness can come to reflect transcendental consciousness beginning to come alive in us. Thus, in coming to know ourselves no longer through a glass darkly, but now face to face, we are the universe coming to know itself consciously fulfilling the entire cosmic becoming.

Now, because life is immortal or at least perennial in the intermediate term transcendental consciousness is not confined to the mortality of any single individual but can become manifest in each and every one of us in so far as we enter into the grail state. Moreover transcendental conscious may in principle be eternal in the same sense that space-time is eternal and may have a cumulative capacity to become aware of itself through the biota over the epochs. However we need to be very clear. There is no God out there in the skies of in the centre of stars, or in the black holes, or dark wastes of the universe. The only source of transcendental consciousness lies in the biota and God cannot come alive more than we can come alive ourselves in our transcendental experience ad in so doing bring about a beneficent age of conscious enlightenment.

Moreover, although Jesus was a brilliant visionary genius and his teachings, especially in the Gospel of Thomas, are inspired, worshiping Jesus as the Lord and savior, the only begotten Son of God is a complete useless deception and a tragic fallacy that has led to martyrdom,

Crusade and Inquisition. Prayers are also useless except in so far as they help individuals come closer to the centre of cyclone of transcendental consciousness.

Traditional religions rather than fulfilling the unfolding of transcendence, become oppressive and sometimes diabolical social forces mediating militant cultures by asserting moral paradigms which aid internal cooperation to achieve utopian dominion, thus hijacking the actual transcendental consciousness, murdering or exiling the visionaries, from Zechariah to Jesus, and seizing the priesthood in the name of civic order and utopian military dominance. This is a totalitarian social process being driven not by prophetic consciousness or visionary experience but by a priesthood liked to the established order imposing patterns of belief in a moral deity and attitudes which repress women and female reproductive choice for male cultural imperatives.

Jesus was a great visionary, but to turn him into a pagan cypher of himself as a perpetual Greek demi-god hanging dripping with blood on every church pulpit would make him turn in his grave and regret having every pronounced the immanent Kingdom.

Now enters a peculiar disrupting influence, to the rule of diabolical order in the form of the theogenic species, which every culture which has discovered them, despite some being themselves violent warrior cultures, has given sacred and revered status to.

Fortunately, although some of these agents are outright poisonous, we have been blessed with some very potent and yet beneficent transcendental catalysts. Psilocybin for example has an active dose a thousand times smaller than the mean lethal dose and no capacity for addiction. Alcohol by contrast like heroin and paracetamol has a mean lethal dose only some ten times higher than the active dose. Not only that but it is not a drug but a living sacrament like all the food on which we depend for our survival. It is pure and trustworthy and genetically produced.

The basic gist here is that because evolution explores the "phase space" of possibilities, it is next to inevitable that the biosphere will contain species that contain agents that will modulate the sappy biochemical brain in just such a way as to open the doors of perception, so that our ego consciousness suddenly finds itself facing the overwhelming flood tide of a reality that brings all our experiences from dream, memory and reflection into one kaleidoscopic vision of the totality—be it heaven or hell depending on how we see it.

Throughout history some individuals have always been close to the visionary doorway either just because their genes have predisposed their brain chemistry to be close to the edge of 'sanity' (humans vary up to a 100-fold for instance in their monoamine oxidase activity, profoundly affecting their serotonin metabolism). For example William Blake, and even our Liz, share a natural tendency to visionary experience probably shared by Ezekiel and others in former times.

However these visionary and prophetic experiences, sometimes driven by starvation, sensory deprivation, self-abuse, or long desert vigils, far from being more genuine manifestations of a higher consciousness, are generally stereotyped, limited and often frankly paranoid visions of cosmic conflict and violence amid a general trend of seeing the light of God or a vision of the "holy one" with white hair riding on chariots of fire, or the vengeful Lord Jesus condemning a third of the stars and trees to demise because of the vagaries of Nero.

This just leads to a dreadful outcome, in which the major world cultures are deleteriously positioned to cause an apocalyptic hard-landing for humanity, through desert-loving scorched-earth religions, which not only repress women but rape the planet and thus are no antidote to materialistic selfish business as usual which hey claim as the moral high-ground.

Apocalypse is real because human consciousness has a genetic propensity for religious experience through the doors of perception being leaky enough to let in the light of the unveiling, but we are completely ill-equipped to deal constructively with the situation we find ourselves in, leading to planetary damage and the clash of the cultures.

The organic result creeping up on us is that the visionary species do have the power to give us a remarkably safe journey across the Styx, so we can actually come to discover how this whole cosmic becoming actually works, and far from being a shallow or false superficial side show, by comparison with genuine spiritual experience of the so called sages, are our own cosmic destiny coming up to meet us, and the universe's cosmic destiny coming to realize itself too.

Notice the contradiction here between our so called enlightened democratic Western society, which has banned magic mushrooms despite their manifest safety, particularly when used in a protected religious ritual, and two to three thousand years of sacred use by human cultures. And it is most telling that they have been banned without real evidence of harm or danger largely for the very reason that they do open the doors of perception and thus threaten the social order of consumer based Christian culture.

To be even more specific, Christianity is a sacramental religion whose holy communion is sine qua non based on eating the flesh and drinking the blood of the redeemer. This diabolical cannibalistic sacrament is a false sacrament which at best is no more effective spiritually than the mildest tipple and is a false representation of a spiritual communion based on frankly neolithic ideas of sacrificial violence. It s then little wonder and a commentary on the spiritual fragility of Western society that we have sought to ban these agents of genuine enlightenment with severe penalties comparable to Deuteronomy's dire penalties for adultery, parental disobedience or worshipping strange gods rather than find ourselves able to rightly incorporate them into our traditional worship, despite the fact that in all experiments where conventional non drug taking people are given the opportunity, they claim to have genuine religious experiences which remain of beneficial significance and meaning to their lives years later.

*Now let's return to your hopeful monster of far baryons and other hypothetical particles to fix something that ain't broke. The problem is this. Physicists for good reasons hypothesize various kinds of putative particles from axions, through super-symmetric partners like gravitons to dark matter to explain real phenomena (the galaxies remain stable at a rate of rotation which would throw them apart unless there is dark matter), or to complete a meaningful fundamental theory that would better explain the standard model and its unification with gravity (super-symmetry, shadow matter). However, you are coming from a different direct altogether which is trying to turn religious belief in an appealing but fraudulent model of reality into a scientific justification for a created universe in which all thought and evolution is just a shadow play of the creator deity. I guess you feel safer with such a delusion but is it safer really? Aren't we all safer being part of a robust cosmological life process in which life has a central cosmological role of becoming?

You want to try to prove life is created by a fictitious non-evident mythologic deity because you have been indoctrinated by Catholic beliefs. You aren't prepared to accept the clear scientific evidence that life has evolved, but place your faith in a fictitious third party to place a losing bet that life can't sustain its own creative evolution.

You want to use the plethora of hypothetical particles and some even more far fetched fictitious ones like baryonic dark matter to show that, given all these mysterious shadowy possibilities, your mythological fictitious and highly vindictive deity might be pulling the marionette strings of reality to make everything happen and hence make the universe acceptable and meaningful to you. Baryonic dark matter is a misnomer which has no role and is mimicking baryonic ordinary matter when we don't know real dark matter if it exists mirrors ordinary matter in a baryonic way forming quark composites under the weak and strong forces. This is extremely unlikely because you are asking dark matter to behave just like light matter. Moreover there is no role for this interaction in biology.

Now you are right that given the sheer number and variety of exotic particles imagined by various physicists if we really need to have God pulling the marionette strings, we could imagine one or other might be doing the trick. But this is as I said trying to make moonbeams our of cucumbers. It is a mirage that will surely evaporate because the agent God doesn't actually exist and the only particles we will end up finding are those that genuinely make the physical universe and life possible."

Chris

End of Ch. 3

CHAPTER 4

Reply to a Mathematics Professor Comments

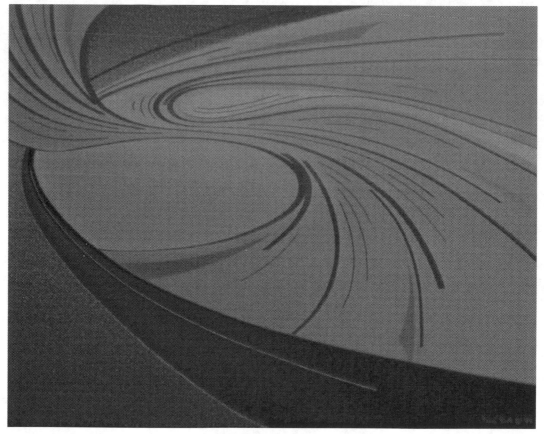

Kinetic Force

—In WEDconscious@yahoogroups.com, "Dhushara" wrote:

"Neural synchrony is (not) about . . . . simultaneity of processing audio-visual input and the verbal linguistic input." Parenthesis added.

Angell: Honestly, I do not understand how any reader can understand my 'Spanglish' ramblings! I am trying to say too many things in one breath. Chris, what you are saying is true but I am trying to emphasize the importance of requiring the joint participation of both the theorist and the practitioner when assessing the real time needs of a patient so that an adequate therapeutic protocol can be designed. It accentuates on the crucial importance of extracting the truthful content of the patient's verbalization of his ailment during that first visit. What we are witnessing is an unfortunate polarization where the clinician, too busy or lazy to update his practice, becomes a local robot repeating that same old treatment and the theorist, unfamiliar or uninterested in the patient needs, becomes the universal robot repeating the same mathematical logic formulas applying to all creatures anywhere in the cosmos. For me to be able to communicate why this problem may be minimized in behalf of a more accurate diagnosis and treatment for any condition at all I need to explain the philosophical basis underlying the problem which means discussing the evolution of complexity so that the possible solution is meaningful and credible.

We have 1) material things (unit dimension, or aggregates thereof), 2) their attributions (color, dimension, form, shape, etc.) and 3) an observer. Since all three can change, we simplify by choosing an unit invariant particle dimension anywhere in cosmos and consider how the potentially variant attributions may influence any observer's account about the physical material truthful state anytime, anywhere. IMO this can be represented by variations on Paul Dirac's mathematical formulation using vector calculus <bra-ket> notation you are familiar with. It contains an invariant component and a variant component affecting the appearance of the invariant, regardless of the presence of any observer anywhere. The complexity is only caused by the 3) observer component. Since our priorities should be concerned with the physical human brain where those material reality variations are encoded in neuronal networks representations, the observer needs to get a truth-content account of the variation as it truthfully happened independent of its appearance to a human observer. This is especially true when the human observer ignores what relevant changes in the assumed invariant material particles may limit or corrupt the sense-phenomenal perceptual input from his internal body proper or external receptors. The interplay between the participating variables may significantly and improperly influence what is really happening to the invariant material brain substrate. Here we have all three components varying in space time and thereby rendering any computational effort to ascertain what is really happening an impossible task, especially if we use rational numbers in the vector analysis and have to reckon with infinities. Thus, we limit the number of variables by assuming the existence of a single invariant quantum material particle state and get falsifiable technological information about the resulting variations from the dynamic interactions of the participating variable elements. Because of my insistence on the priority emphasis on real time verifiable mesoscopic reality as the basis on which to justify flying into conjectures and speculations about what is happening in the physical material brain with no relevant familiarity about its structural and functional aspects, I see the need for the joint presence of the appropriate practitioner and theorist during an evaluation of what is really happening.

Because we humans should be concerned about what is truthfully happening in our brains first before looking into our biosphere and taking theoretical flights of fancy into an unknown cosmos; i.e., we need to know what truthfully is happening in our own brain before we board on that spatial engine. This emphasis on the priority of the human observer's existential reality brings into focus what I consider as being currently ignored by both practitioners and theorists, i.e., how verbal accounts of what is reliably happening in our own material brain may be distorted by the grammatical language structure being used by the reporting patient. I am suggesting how may such probable distorsions of reality may be minimized by substituting the invariant component with the newborn inherited generative grammar (proto-language) and substituting the variable components with the measurable interplay of environmental factors participating at a given moment during a verbal interview.

I discuss how real space-time sense phenomenal perceptual activity comes in three flavors, a graphical audiovisual representation, a putative 'inner language' representation and an unknown brain dark matter source under investigation. The natural neural synchrony of their respective brain matter representation needs further study before the vector analysis can be successfully used.

Hope this clarify my earlier communication ramblings. Angell

*   *   *

Prof. Chris King: "Angell, Neural synchrony is about neural waves of activity that are in phase that is oscillating in synch, not simultaneity of processing audio-visual input and the verbal linguistic input.

The idea is that the in synch excitations distinguish the signal from the groundswell of peripheral activity in various parts of the brain. It's basically a dynamical hologram that can recognize itself. But synchrony itself is the recognizer because the in-synch oscillations naturally reinforce and all the other excitations randomly average out to nothing at all, or next to it, so it all makes perfect sense."

Chris

End of Ch. 4

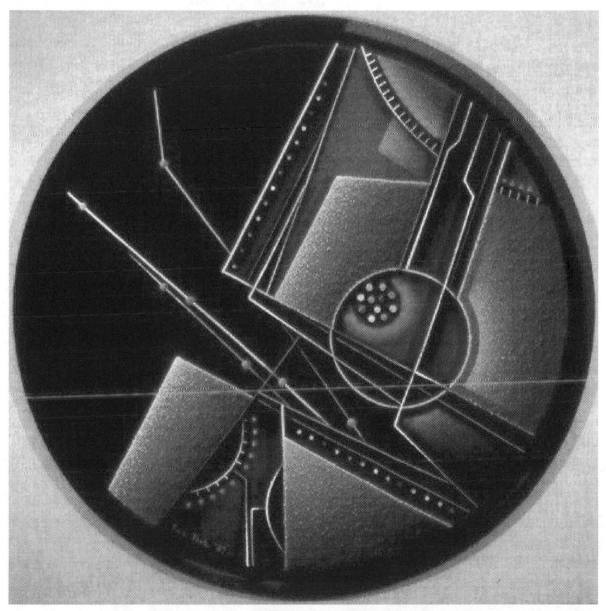

Gamma Activator

INTRODUCTION

To simplify our brief discussion of this most complex theme we are adopting the philosophy doctrine of the excluded middle proposing that the exposition is meaningful and truthful, i.e., sense phenomenal physical descriptions and metaphysical logic explications cannot be simultaneously true and not true because true, consistent, objective, coherent and falsifiable semantic beliefs is the core concept.

Thus one may ask 1) who is the observer transferring the information? ; 2) do we all experience change? 3) is the change experienced linear in its progression? 4) do we all witness the same quotidian existential reality? 5) do we all consistently experience realities that resist being framed into symbols or sentences to ontologically describe or epistemologically explain their meanings? 6) do we all give priority to the biological well being before being concerned with psychic happiness or social acceptance?

Consistent with the doctrine of the excluded middle we find it convenient to use a digital binary code, yes or no. Thus 1) is yes, the observer is always a human being with all the ontological perceptual and/or epistemological conceptual (combinatorial) limitations the human brain consistently exhibits. 2) yes, as consistent recorded history demonstrates. We conveniently epistemologically conceptualized the 'time' function as a measure of change. 3) no, because we all experience recursive cycles in nature, night and day, seasons, etc. Consequently the cycle is not circular but a vortex spiral as it generates a new cycle. 4) no, because existential reality is in the brain dynamics of the beholder where the relative position of the observer in relation to the observed and the internal body proper (neurohumoral) and external information input into the human brain influence the language exposition (language structure) 5) yes, as statistically evidenced in all humans interviews. This experience generates beliefs. 6) no, because recorded history evidences the lives of prophets as behaving against self interest even though the biological imperative drive is in control in the overwhelming majority of the human species as consistently observed. As if our human species were reflexively and subconsciously driven to stay alive as observed even during unconscious sleep states when we track the exact position coordinates of a crawling insect on our face surface before slapping it down. This documented behavior constitutes evidence on the joint participation of both genetically inherited and environmentally acquired control as consistently observed. This behavioral feature we share with evolved subhuman species where the biopsychosocial drive (BPS) is in reflex control.

How do we then reconcile the multiple complex content of interacting variables such as the amount of data, code, text or transfinite radiation input into the dynamic human brain where the information is stored, processed and linguistically or instrumentally transferred as adaptive motor responses to the varying contingencies at play? The short answer is that there cannot be absolute certainty but we can settle for probabilities of occurrence adopting the convenient tools of a probability calculus as refined with Bayesian considerations. Enter quantum theory where we do need to consider the fundamental role played by the instruments used in the measurements that may themselves cause 'entanglements', 'simultaneous ('spooky') control activity at huge distances' and other wonders of creative human activity. Interestingly, in the process the human mind is arriving at a theory of everything (TOE) by adopting a hybrid Epistemontological approach based on the mediation of a mathematical physics vector analysis language using the '<bra-ket>' notation.

ARGUMENTATION

Surprisingly, the evolution of complexity can be equated with the evolution of a quantum theory based on probabilities and its amazing predictive value. It has provided meaning, truth, objectivity and coherence to an otherwise supercomplex and individualized existential reality evolving every instant. Quantum theory is about harmonizing the 'seen and the unseen.' based on their probabilities of being instantiated as an occurrence.

The probability of gaining a deeper and meaningful insight into the workings of nature is predicated upon the real possibility of accessing the information content of a putative closed system with boundaries. If the information sources (objects, events) recede into infinity it becomes inaccessible. Consequently, we need to work with assumed closed systems allowing the observer to precise the temporal course of specific objects/events. This is accomplished by using defined transfinity coordinates for the spatiotemporal location for such objects/ events as substitutes for the unreachable ever receding infinities in a vacuum space. Nature abhors the vacuum. This is accomplished when explicating the properties of a given system by assigning a projection operator for each relevant property in Hilbert Space or subspace thereof. We also need to characterize the spatio-temporal course of events as being not random but stochastic events in nature to statistically assess their many probable behaviors. This way instead of characterizing the spatio-temporal unit evolution of a system as preceding its measurement and collapse, we now assign a Schrodinger function to each coexisting individualized event. For this conceptualization to work it is necessary to assume a linear, time ordered sequence of events so that the projection operators on a tensor product can be mathematically transformed into additions. Besides, only those objects/events that may be assigned the probabilities of 2n possible outcomes can be given a physical interpretation so that it supports the required Boolean algebra. The particular state of a system in space time, when each relevant variable is individualized, is conceptualized as the evolving trajectory of a point singularity in phase space with independent and exclusive, albeit interactive existence in a coarse grained phase space containing varying subsets of arbitrary sized cells. Applying the binary code again, when a given cell has a value 1 it means the singularity point is inside the cell in question or not (value 0) where Bi and Bj indexes these cells such that the integral sum of Bi = 1 and the product BiBj = alpha ij Bj represent the spatio-temporal evolution of the complex system. The metaphysical logic analysis requires that this tensor product of the successive phase spaces be conceptualized as having a volume with an a priori probability of 1. However quantum theory conveniently requires the use of Hilbert Spaces instead of phase space in order to individualize each variable and evaluate their relevant interactions.

The spatio-temporal evolutionary time arrow progression of a complex system from t1 → t2 can best be represented using Heisenberg orthogonal projection operators, the mathematical notations details of which (P(t) = e{Ht P(t0) e•{Ht:) is beyond the scope of this brief essay. Suffice it to say that the orthogonal representation allows for the assignment of probable relevance and weight of a calculation result. The weight of a linear progression between two points in space time is represented as their tensor product mathematically transformed into additions of their phase states histories. It also allows, in our opinion, to structure observations in terms of a time-independent reference invariant state as being influenced in its 'perception' by an observer by the interactivity of the various variant relevant states interacting. While we always try to consistently distinguish the ontological perceptual from the epistemological conceptual, it should be always noted that the phenomenological denotes appearance of particulate matter and its attributions whether measured or inferred by the consistent predictable signature of its presence in real time.

But existential reality is not exclusively linear as, experienced, it has a cyclical recursive component that cannot be ignored. Therefore we need to assume that the human brain linearizes the information input so it can reach the appropriate processing brain neuronal networks. Unfortunately a consistently reliable, credible fundamental biopsychosocial (BPS) model theory of human brain dynamics cannot depend exclusively on a 'measurement interpretation' and we need to assume/conceptualize the hybrid co-existence of real and virtual processes. We anticipate major problems in marketing our speculation on the existence of dark baryonic bosons DNA/RNA receptors because the phase space may be coarse-grained and dividing it into a set of individualized cells of arbitrary size that are mutually exclusive and jointly exhaustive may constitute a mathematical intractable nightmare. Furthermore, the long range goal of our BPS model of brain dynamics becoming a fundamental theory of everything (TOE) cannot rest exclusively on measurement-based interpretations that restricts its reach beyond the mathematical formalism of experimental physics. So much for the current fanciful attempts to cajole quotidian existential reality within the confines of the probabilities generated by artificial intelligence 'algorithmic complexity models', i.e., robotizing human true reality leaving out anything irreducible to language representations such as ethical and moral considerations, affect or the belief in transfinite sources of relevant information causally efficient in controlling human biopsychosocial (BPS) equilibrium. Thus is our concern when calling for the joint presence of the 'hands on' psychotherapist and the 'arm chair theorist' to partake jointly in the evaluation of the underlying brain pathologies as narrated in the expressed language structure of the patient. The truth content of an underlying pathology can be manipulated in any medium whether expressed in symbols, sentential logic or a garden variety language structure.

On the other hand if you dream about a BPS fundamental TOE then there are two important elements to take into consideration: the relation between an underlying theory framework and quantum / Bayesian conditioning logic reasoning; the framework invisible rules should not only be convenient but also relevant and compatible as a minimum. In our case, as briefly noted above, it requires the tensor products of the sets of 2-d subspaces projected into Hilbert space—as amended by Wheeler's theoretical 'delayed response' in transactional exchanges—to accommodate the experimental wave/particle superposition of states as recorded by the grid interferometer detector results. Intuition may become a poor resource in guiding quantum mechanic's experimental designs ("spooky actions at a distance").

It is to be noted how the von Neumann approach is taking the distinctive **results** of quantum **measurements** as its point of departure for developing the formalism 'after the fact' without taking into account the previous state of the system preceding the measurement. Needless to say that macro cosmology and micro sub Planckian micro states both require a closed system approach and need to be reconciled before quantum gravity and the conjecture we make about a dark baryonic polynucleotide receptor takes hold as the putative link between a transfinite source and the human brain neocortical pre-motor phase space acceptor.

But, absent information about the preceding events before the measurement that collapsed the wave function gives us the opportunity to model a fundamental BPS TOE approach if we split the Schrodinger wave function into two inseparable parts, one representing an invariant system and the other representing the variant, interacting environmental circumstances R(t) that may deceptively modify the perceptual evaluation of the invariant element. It should be noted that the Schrodinger function itself does not generate a binary code element and needs to be complemented with a density matrix element. This we do by adopting the Dirac analytic tool expressed in <bra-ket> notation, as published elsewhere. The meta-verse and a thermal bath vat housing a living brain both may qualify as the 'environmental circumstance'. This approach is necessary to minimize the number of relevant and necessary variables and, while insufficient to deduct such quasi-deterministic detailed laws from first principles, it minimizes the operational conumdrum of handling so many variant, interactive complexities as they evolve from state to state in space time. This way, the invariant of coarse grain in the macro domain of discourse having the largest probabilities are those ascertainable with the classical equations of motion making the goal of decoherence more probable thereby minimizing deviations from those predictions based on their measurements. Operationally it makes it easier to distinguish the individuality of the summed over (tensor products) participating variables causing decoherent distorsions (noise, interference, dissipation, etc) in the phenomenological evaluation. By trading off with the appropriate analog equations of motion, hydrodynamics, energy, momentum or other conserved quantities variables, we can couple/link better with the elusive features of the successful quantum theoretical micro sub-Planckian domain until we achieve their formal reconciliation. Keeping in mind the absolute truth content feature as the guiding goal in the analysis, the main barrier to a reconciliation is that a mixture of interacting quantum states modified in its expressions by the environmental circumstances, tags different probabilities to the participating components and the actual features of the instrument conducting the measurement selects only one of many possibilities as expressed by, e.g., the resulting signatures as tracks, ionization patterns, bubbles, frictional heat dissipation, etc. or, in the case of human language semantic syntax structure, as reports plagued with subconscious confabulations, lies and other distortions/ deviations from the truthful etiology. Without a shared language there is no way to distinguish what is the case from what is thought to be the case. As it turns out, quantum theory probabilistic calculus has provided the most reliable scientific methodology so far. Maybe this is the end of the line for the human mind to scrutinize the relevant but invisible features of our existential reality.

SUMMARY AND CONCLUSIONS

This essay aims at providing arguments for the adoption of the Epistemontological hybrid biopsychosocial BPS model of brain dynamics, as extended, to satisfy the requirements to be considered as a fundamental theory of everything TOE pertaining to the mesoscopic domain of human existential reality in general. Specifically it emphasizes the importance of how, in the author's opinion, understanding how the unavoidable evolution of complexity modifies our phenomenological perception of our own human existence in this 21st. century. At the forefront comes the ontological aspect of our model especially when under the overwhelming pressure of the radical branch of the physicalist reductionist persuasion trying to restrict epistemological cognitive analysis to scientific methodological tools based exclusively on ontological valuations of the truth value content derived from allegedly 'objective' measurements assigning quantitative values to the properties measured while deliberately excluding metaphysical ingredients of crucial and important relevance. This should not to be construed as an 'ab initio' rejection of the Von Neumann model of reality or the Copenhagen standard approach. On the contrary, in our hybrid model they constitute the necessary and most reliable interpretation of the macro world of deterministic classical physics as compared to the quasi-deterministic nature of the quantum theoretical domain of spooky conjectures and speculations albeit their impressive success in their behavioral predictions of systems beyond sensory threshold in the micro sub-Planckian and the macro cosmological domain. Our BPS focus is situated in between both extremes of the reality spectrum, at the mesoscopic level of organization where assigning a value to a measured property means that the property posseses such value as falsifiably, consistently and coherently documented by all observers at all times. This pragmatic approach is well suited as the starting point of a more detailed investigation at all levels. This strategy has applied to the quantum interpretation of reality. But we should continue in search of the defining structure/function of relevant invisibilities beyond the audiovisual or instrumental threshold level value of detection. Ultimately, the attribution of properties to a system is true if and only if, ontologically their probabilities of occurrence must correlate to objective and intrinsic properties of the physical systems being considered. What is truth? Are qualia real? If, as Von Newman suggests, the truth content depends on the measure instrument used, how can anyone epistemologically represent a particular instrument? Absolute truth is in the brain of the beholder.

Because of our model's mesoscopic focus, Tarsky's characterization of the truth value of propositions as being controlled by underlying subconscious mental states especially when expressed in languages with different syntax structures, is routinely validated in the real world. The abstract human being does not exist independent of his individualized circumstance that follows him like his shadow. Language codes for the circumstantial brain representations that guide behavior and the incorporation of knowledge about self, others and the environment. A predominantly subconscious, routine, reflex life style in the majority of the human often impedes the distinction between false and true beliefs. This is especially so when, paradoxically, both may consciously coexist!

Finally, those members of the physicalist faith who exclusively and blindly rely on mathematical physics reductions of reality should be reminded that their commitment to the truth of a scientific claim anchored on statistical surveys, a measurement or a metaphysical logic deduction implies tacit acceptance of all aspects of the underlying framework, data collection, adequacy of the measure instrument, etc. where many aspects are epistemologically irreducible or ontologically defective. So much for scientific methodology skepticism. We suggest again an Epistemontological hybrid approach integrating classic and quantum theoretical perspectives when in harmony with the ongoing orthodox interpretation of real time existential reality such that the amount of data, the code or text that is stored, transferred, received or modified by the relevant medium is accounted for in the final result.

REFERENCES

1) http://philsci-archive.pitt.edu/4549/2/FinalCH.pdf
2) http://plato.stanford.edu/entries/information/supplement.html
3) Blog site: http://angelldls.wordpress.com/;

Dr. Angell O. de la Sierra, Esq.
In Deltona, Florida Winter 2013

End of Ch. 5

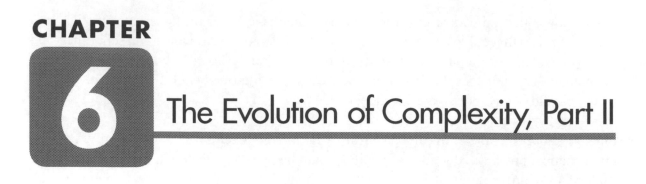

6 The Evolution of Complexity, Part II

Leibniz Monadology From a BPS Model Perspective

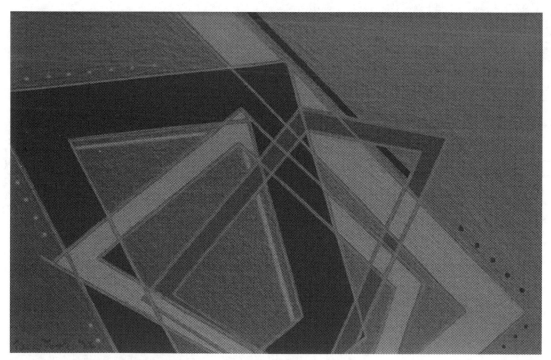

MRS 2095 AD

INTRODUCTION

Leibniz, probably the best mathematician-philosopher in history, in our opinion, unnecessarily wrestled three centuries ago with the perceptual and the conceptual aspects of existential reality, what we have termed the ontological and the epistemological sides of one and the same coin. He ignored that his narrative account is unavoidably a human species version conditioned in its absolute truth content by the phenomenological resolution limits of the human species and the related species limitations in its innate combinatorial capacities to infer the probable structure function of everything relevant but beyond the threshold of being adequately represented for metaphysical logic analysis. Why must his physical brain 'res cogitans' assume that 'attributions' like dimensional 'res extensa' can exist independent of a real material particle beyond the human capacity to measure it? Is it more credible to posit counterintuitive conjectures/speculations than to admit our human brain limitations and market our poem of existential reality as just what it is, an evolving Epistemontological hybrid complexity witnessed as experienced by our limited human brain and narrated when its content is conditioned to the quantum theoretical/Bayesian logic probability of its occurrence. After all, the human narrator, with its uniqueness and limitations, is at the center of the universe transmitting to other humans the most credible account of his mesoscopic reality. Many times we need to prioritize the probable truth content of our models over the elegant esthetic beauty of its narrative content. Keep in mind that the redness of an apple cannot have a phenomenological independent existence, without the material aggregation of unit dimensional— but invisible—particulate matter that made the apple dimensions within the threshold of our human brain sense-perceptual reach. Likewise there cannot be a carrier wave or field without a material particle(s) to be carried. There is a force because there is a particle mass in motion. There is density because matter particles are distributed inside a volume.

Unfortunately neither Feynman, Descartes nor Kant were contemporaneous with Leibniz. Where that unit dimensional physical particle (s) originates has been the subject of many beautiful poems across the ages of recorded history, Big Bang, theological models of creation, self creating and evolving reality faith in physicalist cults, etc. As long as there is a beautiful woman, there will be good or bad poetry depending on its verifiable, falsifiable, and consistent predictability by all observers in the same spatio-temporal coordinates (hopefully to neutralize the Einstein relativistic issues).

It is perhaps time that theorists and scientists alike start seriously discerning the representational map from the measured territory, the conceptual from the perceptual, the mental from the sense phenomenal. And stop thinking about things coming into existence in a 'vacuum' out of 'nothingness', it makes elegant poetry but nature abhors the vacuum! On the other end of the argument, limited as our brains are, why should we discard the probability of these poems? But some poems are more credible than others as we try again to briefly argue in favor of variations on the Dirac formalism of the invariant and interacting variants and how they influence our perceptual perspective as we further blur its absolute truth content when narrating it in our adopted language as detailed before elsewhere.

ARGUMENTATION

The more things change, the more they stay the same, it seems. Scientific and philosophical specialties seem to evolve by 'knowing' more and more about less and less until they approach the asymptotic theoretical limit of knowing everything about nothing! It is irresponsible for evolving nations to **exclusively** dream poems about multi-verses and then consciously ignore the real needs for immediate solutions about health and human suffering in their midst . . . . , and in general. But it may also be as irresponsible when humans become exclusively concerned about their biological health and psycho-social needs, just 'existing' like the evolved members of the subhuman species pack. Most people, admittedly, must limit their contribution to improve on the environmental conditions they found when born on their inherited and acquired resources thereafter. What may be wrong is when those blessed with the advantages of a good superior education feel no conscious responsibility other than self interest conveniences. In that respect they live like a sophisticated subhuman species, totally oblivious of their ethical and moral responsibilities towards the less privileged biosphere neighbors. This becomes all justified, as claimed, under the aegis of a misunderstood individual freedom and libertarianism.

A monad need not be conceptualized in terms of a unit non-dimensional singularity, as a **changing** 'physical' reality experiencing a progression in space time while, in addition, it is simultaneously being subject to undergoing environmental changes, unless you can manage intractable computations leading nowhere. It perhaps makes more sense to conceptualize the unit singularity as an invariant, unit dimensional physical particle where the circumstantial and interacting environmental variables around constitute the variant elements (e.g., particle aggregations and their corresponding attributions in form, size, etc) that are responsible for the human physical brain to possibly experience perceptual errors as to the particle aggregates reality in se.

In our opinion, some self serving theoretical physicists have confused the unit dimensional monad particle with aggregates thereof, the micro sub-atomic Planck unit with the macro cosmology aggregates. It is the latter that is subjected to changing variations as controlled by coexisting environmental complex interactions. These variations are both objective and reliable substantive in appearance but only when appraised by 'normal' observers. As often repeated, there are at times honest and unsuspectingly biased or diseased observers reporting in a foreign adopted language with a significantly different grammatical structure that influences the measured/experienced truth content of the object/event being analyzed. This means that change is not intrinsic to unit dimensional monads as the 'dynamic description' of 'modes' in modern physics would lead you to believe. This statement is, unfortunately conditioned to all observers being situated in the same spatiotemporal coordinates to neutralize relativistic effects. The dynamic behavior of the aggregates may dynamically change but not the monad in our BPS variation perspective. It is always more credible to assume as more logically probable the real existence of helical structures albeit their perceptual invisibility than to expect the student to believe in a domain where opposite-handed helices have only convenient virtual and un-substantive existence. The perceptual mirror reflection of an object is only virtual as to the structure/function performance of the reflection but very real in its phenomenological objective presence.

There cannot be monads not carrying unit dimensional matter particles that progress internally, only aggregates can do so as a function of causally efficient environmental factors, locally and universal in space-time. Only aggregates progression has something to do with perceptions. The individualized parameters of the probable progression in space-time are determined by their path as modified by environmental causality factors both local and transfinitely. The initial and final state of a monad as such is invariant, as argued.

Following the suggestion of philosopher Arthur North Whitehead, we can analogize by considering the human being at conception 'in utero' as being 'tabula rasa' and its cognitive evolution starting by incorporating genetic data from both parents and acquired data from the uterine environment. At that fleeting moment in space-time we may conceptualize an invariant human monad equivalent ready to start its evolutionary path as soon as the fertilized ovum divides. From then on sense phenomenal perceptual input into the developing human brain may be mechanically described/explained on mechanical grounds and corroborated with modern fMRI and EEG measurements. We may, as Feynman stresses, rely almost exclusively on the measured or consistenly observed results depending on the language maturity of the subject and developmental age. His cognitive path into adulthood becomes a function of his genetic/acquired data base content and evidenced as operant conditioning Skinnerian and/ or Freudian behavior or combinations thereof. Here again, we need not confuse the monistic material with pluralistic 'spiritual' that Leibniz's 'graded panexperientialism' struggled with or the 'heterogeneity of modes' modern mathematical theorists dream about.

Within the context of our biopsychosocial (BPS) model of brain dynamics, the invariant 'enduring substance' stem cell represent the human monad equivalent iff we accept the Lamarckian concept that DNA carries along environmental information about yesteryears. Consequently a human monad equivalent carries a genetic/acquired past in the present and the future course of evolution of their dividing aggregates will be determined by internal neurohumoral and external environmental variables. However, considering the loud objection of the physicalist faith adherents regarding Leibniz premises on the required existence of a 'higher order consciousness' intelligent design albeit his deliberate goal of restricting his analysis to mathematical logic, we can only comment that if the materialist wish to rest their case about self-evident cosmological and subPlankian order on the basis of the adequacy of their self organizing/self creating poem and want to violate natural laws of physics in the process, that is their conscious choice. Leibniz explicitly recognized the superiority of animals heightened phenomenological perceptions thus implying that the human brain needs 'further assistance' about 'necessary and eternal truths'. By suggesting a mathematical logic based sub-model about a reciprocal information transfer with transfinite coordinates in space-time via dark baryonic DNA/RNA receptors, we may be answering Leibniz and providing a putative source of survival information for humans across generations. Theological faith can also be reasoned. Interestingly, Leibniz recognizes that existential reality is in the brain of the beholder ('human nexus'). He also recognized the innate limitations on his ontological sense phenomenal acuity and his epistemological capacity to make adequate symbolic/sentential language representations.

However, operationally Leibniz ignores the 'human nexus' and emphasizes more on the epistemological element of a hybrid existential reality. It should also be noticed the exclusively human attribute of being able to introspectively reflect and discover the difference between the "I" and the "other". Leibniz seems to prefer the doctrine of the excluded middle when he suggests the true-false binary code analytical approach. Notably, he accepts that some knowledge may escape human cognition. In reality both ontological and epistemological 'truths' are contingent on the phenomenological acuity and an objective and unbiased metaphysical logic analysis free—when possible—from framework perspective restrictions. The truth content of consistent and falsifiable predictions from cognitive results are as reliable as the axioms, postulates or primary principles on which they rest.

Arguably, one may defend theosophical predictions along same lines of argument as we do when assuming the appropriateness of using a quantum theoretical analysis of probabilities of occurrence. But we are not prepared to sustain, with Leibniz, that the opposite of such propositions are necessarily impossible. This especially so if we necessarily want to avoid inaccessible infinities and have to operationally limit the number of related variable at play, i.e., we have to settle for a proximate, apparent final causality by acknowledging human brain combinatorial complexity and accepting a unit dimensional physical particle or 'grain' as a probable fact. Reality for the human brain must ultimately be the same at the cosmological or subatomic level of organization. This is another argument in favor of having an invariant unit-dimensional physical particle followed by a series of n number of relevant variant and interacting contingencies which we must limit to n-1 transfinities or just the very few elements in the series by approximations. This is part of our proposed Dirac method when subject to a vector analysis. A careful analysis of Leibniz theoretical inferential projections, as opposed to his operational conclusions, indicates his convictions that the phenomenological and the metaphysical are two sides of the same coin, aka the Epistemontological hybrid existential reality. The credibility of this approach should be advanced when quantum theoretical and general relativistic models are reconciled and a reciprocal information transfer between neocortex premotor brain attractor phase space and transfinity is experimentally or logically documented. Informed intuitions almost drive you to suspect that all events in nature are interconnected and a dynamic symmetry may be a goal as opposed to a given, associated with providing a stable and propitious environment for the human species to survive. The symmetry framework goal implies a negentropic violation of a natural law dictum that systems spontaneously evolve to a more stable minimum free energy configuration. But the dynamic order is witnessed and probably responds to transfinite forces in operation for a master universal plan we all strain to reason out but beyond cognitive reach. Should an universe-God replace individual Gods, a la Spinoza? In our BPS model super symmetry is a requirement to justify the important role of gravitons to mediate human information transfer to and from transfinity to reach which God . . . . , an 'a priori' universal God from which the JudeoChrIslamic 'a posteriori' Gods evolved? Once again, we posit that it may be possible to consider an universal God invariant subjected to variants in the way humans vitally 'experience' its 'presence' as conditioned, modified and influenced by the ever changing evolution of existential environmental realities in the biosphere. This experience is then modified further by the individualized observer as he consciously, freely make choices of the best adaptive response to challenges in the existing biopsychosocial (BPS) equilibrium (derivative human 'monads?). The alternative interpretation favored by mathematical theorists, i.e., a self-sustained, generating and evolving causal dynamics progression interpretation, will imply a spontaneous negentropic evolution of complexity and other contrived 'behavior' of charges, etc. that remains like an article of faith contrary to human experience and the physical laws of nature as we now interpret them. It is a tribute to human intelligence to conceptually create such elegant model poems but they leave too many questions un-answered because it leaves out the human brain dynamics factor. We insist that our human theological model of historical biopsychosocial equilibrium that guarantees the survival of the species across generations can be reinforced with metaphysical logic arguments, a sort of Wills's "Grace Based on Reason." if you will. Personally this author emotionally feels as if ultimately, humans are trying to 'restore' the universal God Monad symmetry invariance based on our back-up genetic and acquired memory storage but, once having controlled the emotional bias religious default, metaphysical logic reasoning tells me that before progressing towards a more perfect world as a goal, man has to be alive, happy and psico-socially accepted in his 'pack' because this progression is the exclusive work of our human species, cannot leave it to ants, roaches or Rhesus monkeys to carry the baton trans-generationally! Leibniz in his transcendental genius distinguished the 'passive' from the 'active' but had an ingrained bias toward the epistemological giving low priority to the ontological sense-phenomenal human in his real 4d space-time existence. In our own poem, the 'passive' becomes the invariant monad and the 'active' becomes the multitude of complex variants influencing the perception or distortion of the invariant truth. Unfortunately our current theorists have same bias trying to replace physical particulate matter with their contingent attributions like forces (f=ma) or spontaneous self sustained organized activities. The individualization of an invariant monadic universe gives rise to the variable 'multiverse' concept. This recognizes that there are competing strategies for adaptive success in a particular environment. In the anthropic universe of human mesoscopic reality this individualization usually takes the form of 'prefab' alternatives coexisting in attractor phase space premotor neocortex area of the brain. A freely willed conscious choice depends on humans' immediate and transcendental goals on the basis of its fitness, as exhaustively argued elsewhere. Because humans are the observers, actors and narrators of reality, our cognitive capacities are constrained to the very specific parameters that define human ontological and epistemological limits. This is our human story and every species follows or goes on with their subhuman ways.

Because only humans are the 'language' narrators of existential reality, the narrative has to be understood within the context of humans' inherent and acquired limitations. Consequently, we can only access the probabilities of that invariant universal monad by writing poems about Big or smaller bangs and invent a finite universe where mass, energy, momentum, etc are conserved (cosmological constant) and then hope that our measurements and logic analysis make consistent predictions.

Amazingly, Leibniz's vision in the 18th. century already predicted reciprocal information transfers at ". . . any distance, however great." This includes the constant radiation piercing our atmospheric shield and entering into our phenomenological domain, as if to emphasize the universal interconnectedness. This becomes the basis for our model of reciprocal information transfer from transfinite sources via bark baryonic receptors in DNA/RNA neocortical sites subjected to constant transfinite radiation activity, as mentioned. Fortunately, a quantum probability calculus and a general relativity theory were also invented providing for an universe with no absolute boundaries and we can always tackle infinities with no edges in sight by limiting the number of complex interacting variables participating at will taking into consideration the individualized coordinates metrics in space-time of the instrumental/ human observer. Who could ask for anything more? . . .

As Leibniz elaborates further on his 'evolution of complexity' and finally realizes that the human monad is much more complex to explain there is noted a fundamental shift away from considering a unit-dimensional physical particle as the invariant element in a spatio-temporal progression and settles for shifting brain dynamic patterns without understanding the structure/function basics of brain architecture as most mathematical theorists do today. This biased emphasis on the epistemological is what produces the paradoxes and confusions as Leibniz tries to explain the evolution of his contrived complexity version in humans but operationally leaving him out of the picture. It is proper for Leibniz to continuously modify his model of reality in the light of new scientific developments which excluded the structure/ function details of the human brain as is common even today among mathematical theorists of 'modern' physics who rather exclusively dream of substituting transient 'modes' for particulate matter involving fields, photons, phonons, electron orbitals and other attributions of physical particles without a physical substrate carrier. Good luck! We can always look at the skies but with our feet resting on real solid ground, 'ad astra per asperas'. This is not to deny the importance of justifying the human monad strategy in terms of real time, ongoing quotidian existential ends and means available but also in terms of final causes which this author emphasizes is directed at maintaining the human species survival across future generations via a continuous adjustment of his biopsychosocial (BPS) adaptive equilibrium with his changing environment because reality is in the physical brain dynamics of the beholder, no brain no reality to narrate. If the mathematical theorists leave no room for the psycho-social/psycho-physical parallel models the human race is doomed to disappear in a few generations. Watch out the ants and roaches are coming yonder . . . . !

In this brief account on the evolution of Leibniz monads there is no room for the development of the Dirac vector model variations we have developed. We will follow up in another discussion.

SUMMARY AND CONCLUSIONS

More than three centuries after the mathematical genius of Leibniz made remarkable prescient projections into our ongoing reality we have pointed out how contemporary mathematical theorists continue to market the biased epistemological, metaphysical logic interpretation of existential reality. They have conveniently ignored the remarkable reinterpretation of Leibniz projections by Kant in his classic "Critique of Pure Reason". They have ignored the strictly ontological warnings about the importance of consistent, falsifiable measurements or observation results as the proper beginning antecedent of metaphysical logic speculations on probabilities, important as pure conceptualizations have turned out to be. Physical theorists have conveniently underplay the ontological contributions of Skinnerian operant conditioning behaviorism or Feynman's real time diagrams representations or Freudian psychology or the psycho-physical parallel approach to ontological phenomenological reality, the Penrose-Hameroff model or even Voltaire's misguided existentialism. Why ignore it, why not team up with experienced psychotherapy practitioners? Those who have not learned the lessons of history are doomed to repeat it as Will Durant warned. Leibniz had valid excuses to de-emphasize or ignore altogether what we have learned after he died in the 18th. century about brain dynamics research and had to be biased in favor of metaphysical, mathematical logic which he was more familiar with. There is no excuse now to continue ignoring the relevance of human brain dynamics as part and parcel of any mathematic analysis poem. Why would, otherwise privileged, mathematical minds insist on giving more importance to the red color attribution of an apple ignoring the physical particulate matter that made it possible? Why not accept the Leibniz projection that progression into an ordered structure "would not occur spontaneously from a simple bird's nest to a cathedral" Furthermore, why should a code of human ethics and morality (as argued by Kant) should be considered irrelevant to a 'physical dynamics' human account of existential reality? Go figure! Will somebody out there explain itto them?

REFERENCES

1) http://www.ucl.ac.uk/jonathan—edwards
2) Blog site: http://angelldls.wordpress.com/;
3) Family Domain site: http://delaSierra-Sheffer.net

Dr. Angell O. de la Sierra, Esq.
Early Spring 2013-04-05 Deltona, Florida

End of Ch. 6

 Epistemontological Synthesis of Psychopathological States, Part I

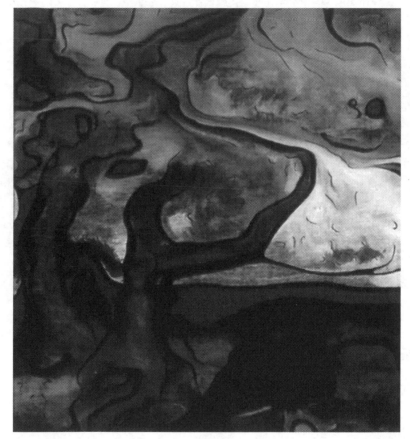

Turbulence

INTRODUCTION

According to the current 'practice of psychiatry' one often wonders why should psychiatrists be required to have a medical degree where training emphasis is made on the molecular, cellular, histological and organ level and their phenomenological 'observed' neurobiological variations in a physical brain leading to measured behavioral malfunction? The current symptomatic handling thereby makes no commitment as to the underlying causes of mental illness. After all psychopathology is an account of bodily processes especially in, but not restricted to, the morbid anatomy of the brain, i.e., no brain no mind! Why restrict the understanding of such body processes to first person narratives where patient confabulation may blur the real causal dynamics of the underlying processes?

On the other end of the diagnostic spectrum we find those unfamiliar with the physical human brain cyto-architecture using diagnostic physio-pathologic labels as convenient heuristics to compose a metaphysical model poem of brain dynamics. Neither the exclusive ontologically based scientific methodology of the current practice nor the exclusive epistemological symbolic and/or sentential representations of metaphysical logic will do. We need to hybridize the perceptual phenomenology with the conceptual and inferential to get the optimal results. To fix our car we prefer to have the most experienced hands-on mechanic 'practitioner' of the 'how' than can apply the latest technological understanding of the relevant theoretical physics applicable to predict and explain the most probable 'what', 'when', and 'where' is the causal agency of the car malfunction. We deliberately leave aside what we consider the most important element controlling the trans-generational survival of the human species, i.e. metalogic 'why' as yet another level of understanding. In what follows we attempt to synthesize both extreme approaches as one unit whole in dealing with the unit whole brain in its different manifestations.

ARGUMENTATION

Should psychiatry be considered 'exclusively' as a theory driven classification, cognitive neuroscience effort providing an objective understanding of mental illness? Or as a 'practice' where the identification of symptoms to particular pathologies as departures from normal function exclusively define brain disease and its pragmatic, empirically-based therapeutic handling? We think that, because of its complexity, both aspects should be handled as a team effort of subspecialists. An accurate prediction rooted on objective and accurate phenomenological measurements resulting in a causally efficient identification of the culprit and its effective control should guide any attempt to restore and improve on the human species biopsychosocial equilibrium, as defined elsewhere http://delaSierra-Sheffer.net. It is true that the metaphysical logic models' speculations with high probability of certainty only provide a convincing heuristic poem for further etiological enquiry into the quasi objective identification of causally efficient factors but—if reliable—it adds another dimension in our knowledge of the health problem to be resolved. A case in point is to include in the diagnosis the relevant role that the genetic and environmental—external and body proper—influences and their causal interactions may play in the quotidian existential coping with ongoing reality. Eric Kandel already recognizes in his molecular reductionism view of psychiatry that the symptoms of mental illness involve both the disruption of biological and cognitive processes without elaborating. However most of these modern reductionist approaches are premised exclusively on viewing the brain as a digital computer carrying out the symbolic or sentential representations to develop algorithms to carry out a programmed goal. We believe there is still much more to brain dynamics than the execution of information processing tasks. Multilevel approaches should not be construed as multiple etiological causations. We gain more by considering mental illness as one cause with multiple manifestations. On the classical practice end of the spectrum the exclusive reliance on the phenomenological symptoms, signs and morbid pathology assumes certainty and transparency in what the specific causation is. While we emphasize in our biopsychosocial (BPS) model the importance of reliable and falsifiable information input and the excesses of self serving epistemological model poems, we'd rather question that phenomenological certainty and empirical adequacy strategy and rather settle for a 'triage' strategy leaving room for the quasi determinism of quantum probabilities and other statistical methods. It is not that simple when we have to reconcile two coexisting conscious views of the same reality as expanded on in Volume V of our series on Neurophilosophy of Consciousness where we distinguish the coexisting conscious realization that we have simultaneously at our disposal in the decision-making process both a metaphysical, rational 'pathogenic' and a material physics-based 'patho-plastic' choice—as amply discussed elsewhere—as often giving rise to situations where contrasting choices between being driven by emotions (related to plasticity of me and my personal existential circumstance) or driven by a rational logic model poem causes ambivalence and confusion, to say the least. It is the latter mental state that will explain the historically recorded cases of altruistic acts against self bps equilibrium interests as experienced by the historical prophets in the JudeoChrIslamic tradition. Furthermore, from a philosophical point of view, why be content with saving the human species until evolution brings in the next successful species to replace us? We are here to stay as the supreme species by adopting adaptive strategies to harmonize with the constantly evolving/changing environment. Recorded human history is our best witness in the defense of an integrated pluralism where the individualized existential reality can be reduced to a credible model poem that considers what we have in common with evolved subhuman species (BPS adaptive equilibrium) and what distinguishes us as an unique 'creation' to lead the way into the trans-generational evolution destiny, whatever that may be. This 'philosophical psychopathology' strategy is usually derogatorily considered by 'psychiatric practitioners' as irrelevant to their current practice specifically when it had to borrow the rational concept of intentionality (See Fodor) to explain the characteristic disturbances of intentionality and consciousness that characterize mental disorders. In reality both the theosophic and the empirical approach are both ultimately different types of beliefs common to our human species trying to deal with its known ontological perceptual and epistemological conceptual limitations.

Perhaps the most difficult element to understand by the psychiatric practitioner is the relevance of the morality and ethics framework of his patients unless they become aggressive or suicidal. We have almost exhaustively discussed what we considered as the best explanation of this issue, Kant's Critique of Pure Reason because, in our opinion, it represents an integration of the **sensory** based phenomenology and the relevant quotidian, **extrasensory** existential reality. In our BPS model we assigned a priority to the unconscious biological imperatives of life preservation as guiding the subconscious drive to adopt viable psycho-social behavioral strategies. Recognizing that moral judgments are simultaneously guided by rational and affective feelings we understood the importance of an adaptive BPS equilibrium harmony with real time existence, something we share with evolved domesticated subhuman species that stay alive, are happy and like to be convivial as a matter of sheer biological survival. But this would not be enough when trying to explain historically backed altruistic acts of prophets against self interest, i.e., contra natura. So we felt the need to conceptually explain, if not perceptually identify the putative source of righteousness, located somewhere in transfinity spacetime coordinates. After all, we have fairly successful molecular models for autism and other mental aberrations the current psychiatry practitioner won't hear about notwithstanding the dramatic insights into brain dynamics by fMRI and other high tech measurements.

SUMMARY AND CONCLUSIONS

It should be abundantly clear from some of our previous publications on the "Neurophilosophy of Consciousness" that the welfare of the neuropsychiatric patient is of the essence as evidenced by the intervention of the triage personnel during a visit to the Emergency Room to stabilize the patient according to the signs and symptoms and laboratory evidence available. This handling is premised on the assumption that symptomatic treatment according to a standard DSM psychiatric protocol is exclusively all there is to be taken into consideration by the current psychiatry practitioner about the causally efficient elements involved. The complexity of the human being makes any search for etiological causation becomes irrelevant at any other higher cognitive level, notwithstanding the many successes of modern technological measurements that dig deeper into probable causation. This is the difference between certainty based on incomplete and limited information to make lasting judgments and the probability of getting a better defined etiology based on more reliable and falsifiable data at the molecular, cellular, histological and organ. Modern psychopathology should become a team effort because of the complexity of the human patient. It should include both the **static** current practitioner and the **dynamic** theorist for the ultimate welfare of the patient.

- http://delasierra-Sheffer.net

Dr. Angell O. de la Sierra, Esq. In Deltona, Florida Winter 2013

End of Ch. 7

Epistemontological Synthesis of Psychopathological States, Part II

Conflicting Mental Representations of the Same Phenomenological Data

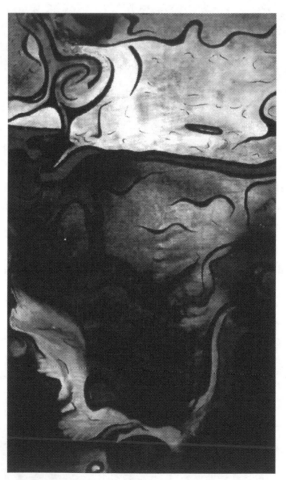

Moor

INTRODUCTION

In our continuing effort to strengthen our previously published arguments on one important conjecture/speculation in the BPS model of brain dynamics premise about the uniqueness of the newborn human proto-language in making possible an adaptive, evolving generation of thought (as expressed in the adopted language), we extend the analysis to discuss how the brain's inherited and acquired information processors join forces in allowing for the adaptive evolution of language in a constantly changing body internal and external environment. We anticipated the logical need for an inherited protolanguage with an essential and unique inner structure capable of keeping pace with changing reality as articulated/expressed in the adopted current language structure. This is the position of the Chomsky neuro-linguists in their defense of an inherited generative grammar as opposed to the Wittgenstein psycholinguists advocating language use as the exclusive causally efficient agency influencing the current language structure by subjecting empirical linguistic input to the general principles of human cognition. We provide arguments for both models and argue for the need of a synthesis of both contrasting models. This synthetic effort includes an attempt to analyze how may audio-visual and verbal inputs can be synchronized into a common brain representation and subjected to a Dirac type vector analysis formulations (<bra-ket> version) with useful predictive value. We also follow up on a previous discussion on how in the process we may also generate a contradictory, self-defective, conscious paradox as evidenced in clinical psycholinguistic assessments, FMRI and EEG data as was briefly singled out in another previous publication. See: http://angelldls.wordpress.com/2013/02/02/controlling-the-self-deceptive-syndrome/

ARGUMENTATION

Language-based mental representations of sense phenomenal physical reality are sensitive to both the human familiarity with the perceptual experience of the variable physical object/event attributions (previously experienced by an invariant brain particulate matter aggregation) and the current language tool ability/competence to generate the corresponding truthful symbolic and/or sentential mental representation. We need not consider either one, the intensional Chomsky or the extensional Wittgenstein models, as exclusive of the other even though admittedly, perceptual information is not as defective as conceptual information truthfulness input can be in the decision-making process.

These considerations brought us early on to the complex conundrum of having to analyze the mind-brain interface by compartmentalizing it into a language $\longleftrightarrow$ thought interface component and a different 'self' $\longleftrightarrow$ language-thought interface separately. To illustrate, after much confusion, we decided to consider the introspective discovery of 'self' as an internal, body proper, indirect perception (different from the classic neuro-humoral environmental input) as different from the 'other' physical things outside. This implied, at the same time, that the paradoxical metaphysical 'self' becomes the driving force behind the co-generation of language and thought! However, this most controversial element of the BPS model, charged with the denotation of 'self', is assisted by the direct confirmation of the different spatiotemporal coordinates of the observer 'I' and the observed 'other'. Notice how this conceptual, universal, invariant physical brain generated the indirect perception of 'self' to distinguish our human uniqueness from other subhuman species. See Dretske, 1999 for a related analysis. This way, the media of information conveyance by the linguistic representation of thoughts becomes dependent on the idiosyncrasies in structural features of the acquired language while the sense phenomenal features become image-like media representations (symbol-filled arrays) of the same experience. The interactive dependence of the graphic phenomenological and the corresponding language-coded metaphysical brain representations is obviously apparent. The conceptualization of a sense phenomenal object/event requires the observer's instantation of the experience as a requisite sine-qua-non to generate phenomenal beliefs. Likewise, you cannot conceptualize phenomenological experiences using language symbolic/sentential tools (e.g., propositions in language of thought) unless the observer personally experienced the audiovisual sensory imaging of the object/event. The challenge of proving that an audiovisual and a discursive content share a common linguistic media of information transfer may never be achieved unless modern technology allows for the synthesis of analog continuous attributions and digital discontinuous core particles components into one common linguistic media for an effective/reliable information transfer role. This alternative is reminiscent of how the measurable invariant, discontinuous, physical particulate nature (digital) remains in inseparable association with the also measurable, varying, continuous, metaphysical wave nature (analog) of its mode of propagation. Is the invariant, discontinuous, material particulate nature of an apple more important than its variable continuous nature of its red color reflections evidencing its ripeness state? Surprisingly, the answer may depend on the individualized conscious choice of the observer! Is that different from the measurable invariant, discontinuous, digital nature of the substrate brain material particles and the also measurable variations in space-time, continuous, analog nature of the particles attributions, e.g., its waveform way of propagation? Is it possible that aggregated brain particulate matter (digital, measurable, invariant and, discontinuous), correlates with the conscious choice of selecting/parsing the analog, variable and continuous language structure that is relevant and appropriate to our true feelings? Are thought representations in neural networks organized like language structures?

In this brief discussion we distinguish the linguistic competence from the performance in the use of an adopted language. Because language generation is the result of a physical brain activity it cannot claim entire independence from other human cognitive processes. The moment a toddler discovers he is different from the sense phenomenal 'other' world within sight or hearing (see Piaget), the process of individuation in language competence starts. His/her ability to learn a language from his parents varies according to inherited factors while performance abilities are acquired and vary according to historic-geographical factors, themselves subject to generational changes or geographical isolations created by mountain ranges or national boundaries. Yet, their internal invariant structure of the brain physical micro substrate is arguably the same, as discussed earlier.

While for Wittgenstein externalists languages are social-historical entities influenced by clear historic-geographical individuation conditions, languages unavoidably also share on the human species' biological individuation process. These underlying biopsychosocial (BPS) equilibrium processes are also present in evolved subhuman species. This underscores the fact that individual human 'BPS' beings and their circumstances cannot be exclusively considered as social groups.

The subtle confusion comes about when both extreme intensional and extensional researchers isolate the common 'BPS' equilibrium needs of the 'idiolect singularity' of their virtual subject of investigation from the equilibrium conveniences of the same individual when adapting to the dialect or language of a geographical, social, historical, or political group. Computer generated I-languages are thus best understood as the 'BPS' brain dynamics properties of the minds of the virtual individuals who know them. Experimentally this requirement has been met when testing the biological endowment of a 'brain in a vat' equivalent isolated from psycho-social environmental circumstances as has been done in retinal vision experiments using modern technologies. To illustrate, identical twins share the same internal states but suppose there exist unknown body-proper visual environmental variations in their quotidian real time existential reality, such as retinal pathology in one of the twins? Have you ever been able to distinguish psychosocial behavioral differences by the twins different choice of syntacto-semantic structure when responding to the same relevant questions during a clinical interview? These studies are well documented by observing the fMRI and EEG parameters during such interviews. The very same external reality causing different mental states as expressed in their language structure conscious choice. See Chomsky, 1995. The real challenge to the intensional/generative grammarians is to formulate a convincing representation/reduction of this conceptualization to show that the extensional truth value arguments in behalf of the psycho-social substratum of all languages is logically false. Instead, the 'intensional' exclusivist interpretation suggest that languages are just convenient variations on a needed theme common to all, the biologically inherited proto-language generative grammar. This interpretation *stresses the need but ignore the BPS conveniences as illustrated by the distinction between the innate competence and the acquired language-based conscious choice of verbalizations, as discussed.

The exclusivist 'intension' argument goes as follows: When we say 'The apple is red we are describing the phenomenological attribution/predicate of the subject apples in general (barring any visual color defects of the observer). This means there is an invariant particulate matter in the brain with a potentially variable attribution of color. As expressed, is this a truth valued reality for all normal human observers anywhere in space time, regardless of their visual physiological facts? Does it matter? The red extensional appearance of the invariant particulate matter in a physical apple is shared by all particulate matter with that same sense-phenomenal redness attribution, not just apples. We don't need to consider now the serious sense-phenomenal limitations of human observers as compared to other sub-human species observing same apple.

If we were to restrict our domain of discourse by moving from the still extensional predicate set of all universal particles of red matter appearance to a consciously chosen predicate sub set of general red apples contained therein, we can still represent the 'intensional' invariant aspects of the apple and the extensional varying aspects of their redness appearance.

By using quantum probabilities and metaphysical logic analysis, we can represent that set—or any other equivalent set—using symbolic/sentential tools. Choosing Dirac's vector space '<bra-ket>' notation as the analytical tool we can explicate the universal invariant aspect of the set in terms of a general mathematical function able to explain more restricted domains as: $f(n) = n \times n$ where 'n' can represent, e.g., either a number sequence (integers2 like 12, 22, 32 . . . n2) or a word sequence (e.g., the word 'apples', 'semantic', 'structures', 'syntax', etc.). The invariant aspect applies to any domain on which the operation 'x' is defined and the variant aspects of any color can be coded. Notice that if the various ways of expressing redness had been formulated as a sequence of 'rational' numbers, it will contain infinity terms that we want to avoid. Each appropriate co-extensional member of the variable set may interact with each other and modify the extensional **appearance** of the universal red apple (e.g., wet, bright, dark, etc.) thus compromising the truth value of the phenomenological visual perception. Let us see now how this reasoning may apply to a language structure.

Any adopted language can be identified with the set of what is common and invariant to ALL languages (inborn generative grammar) and the subset of possible variations in relevant word sequence structure, rhyme, syntax, etc. of the adopted language. The difference between the invariant, intensionalist common universal structure (its generative grammar) and the extensionalist variations of these structural parameters in the adopted language—as empirically experienced during clinical interviews—is at the root of this controversy between intensional and extensional model defenders. In our opinion the intensional model provides for an individuation of linguist expressions making room for the individual and his relevant circumstances regarding his competence and experiences in the use of the language used to report his ailments. The value of Chomsky's mathematical formulation is that it can be a useful analytical tool for many issues besides language.

SUMMARY AND CONCLUSIONS

We hope there should be no doubt about the self-evident fact that a sense phenomenal object or event precedes its symbolic or sentential mental representation and not the other way around. But mental representations are often made of conceptual thoughts with no sense phenomenological features like e.g., qualia. On the other end of the spectrum there are sensations/feelings with clear phenomenal neurohormonal etiological features that resist conceptual strait jackets. Either one or both situations can define a mental state. The same hybrid taxonomy applies to extensionalist expressions of natural languages integrating a physical sensory object/event with a possibly biased belief as to, e.g., its origin. What we can learn from this experience is that, as it turns out, semantics and pragmatics are a central part of the study of any adopted language that preceded the evolution of a newborn inherited proto-language into what currently is considered 'current' in later stages of his development. We do not assign a name to an object/event we have not sensory experienced first. Furthermore, any mind/brain model should try to explain the extensional environmental variations within the context of the intensional brain parameters, Exploring the syntacto-semantic interface will likely remain an unsolvable big challenge indeed unless the issue becomes a shared joined object of investigation between science, philosophy and psychotherapists. We need to integrate the epistemological 'intensional' aspects with the ontological sense-phenomenal aspects as an Epistemontological unit whole. We continue to narrow our domain of discourse by analyzing now the truth value meaning assigned to verbalizations expressed using the language structure of the adopted language.

The same distinctions made in the preceding analyses apply when different extensional expressions in any given natural language about the same reference object/event is observed. This implies that the truth value content expressed in the same given language by two individuals may yet contain different language structures and underlying conceptualizations as Frege underscored, i.e., two individuals linguistically expressing in a given language the same phenomenontological physical reality while having different, but hidden, mental states representations may assign different meanings to the same experience.

To facilitate our pedagogical analysis we preferred to model how an internal and invariant physical brain is influenced by externally varying environmental conditions as expressed linguistically. We consider 'environment' as both the measurable internal body proper neuro humoral milieu and the external measurable/observable varieties and their appropriate mental representations as seen from the perspective of a 'representational theory of mind' in a joint effort to find meaning (semantics) to potentially damaging information inputs to the currently adapted individual BPS equilibrium.

How do we best verbally express in a given acquired language the relations between the invariant physical brain and the mental representations of the internal/external variable physical environment affecting it? We ask the question, what is the truth value of an expressed statement? Could there be present a confabulatory state (illusion, hallucinations, etc.), a self-serving interest or an underlying altruistic intention being expressed? What is the best way to gain an insight into this complexity?

The best model should be able to ontologically describe/identify and/or epistemologically explain the causally efficient agency driving the changes observed, taking into consideration our human species innate perceptual and conceptual brain limitations. Within these limitations we cannot but emphasize the probabilistic nature of both aspects which are currently best described by a quantum theoretical/Bayesian logic approach. Reliable and falsifiable physical measurements / observations with credible metaphysical logic are of the essence. Either isolated component may be necessary but not sufficient to satisfy the important truth value goal. This stresses the need for a dynamic integration as herein suggested.

In our opinion Chomsky's mathematical model approach can be updated to make it possible to extract more meaning from relevant 'invisibilities' escaping phenomenological identification in a predictive way. This way the confusion created by the common paradoxical occurrence of an existing mental representation being caused by a physical object/event that the brain does NOT represent is minimized. To illustrate, the previous mental representation by a toddler of the behavior of a family pet dog, when applied to the unfamiliar sighting event of an escaped wolf from the local zoo may bring disastrous consequences if their sudden unanticipated encounter were to materialize! Identical twins with different behavioral attitudes to the same existential physical reality proves the point. In our quotidian existential reality extensional oriented psychotherapies trump any intensional-oriented approach. A neuro-linguist led analysis of patient expressions describing his ailment may discover etiologies otherwise unavailable to the psychotherapist practitioner charged with the responsibility of saving his life after a putative suicide attempt! Theoretically the extensional act precedes its formulation but in real life a causally unrelated false formulation, illusions, hallucinations, etc. may drive overt or restrained behavior.

The coexistence of conscious awareness of conflicting mental representations is yet another problem we analyzed elsewhere. Unfortunately these considerations do not enjoy wide popularity among the practitioners and are not taken to be of central importance in the design of a causal and content-based psychotherapeutic protocol. In the pursuit of an adaptive BPS equilibrium, most people would subconsciously be driven by acts that make them healthy, happy and socially convivial whether the driving forces are the results of faulty perceptions of causal factors or not. We have emphasized on the crucial importance of mental representations as determined by the dynamic brain properties intrinsic to the patient such as the syntactic structure of his acquired language or his linguistic competence in processing demanding intramental computations or his inferential capacities.

Dr. Angell O. de la Sierra, Esq. In Deltona, Florida Winter 2013

End of Ch. 8

Epistemontological Synthesis of Psycholinguistics and Neurolinguistics. Chomsky vs. Skinner or Both?

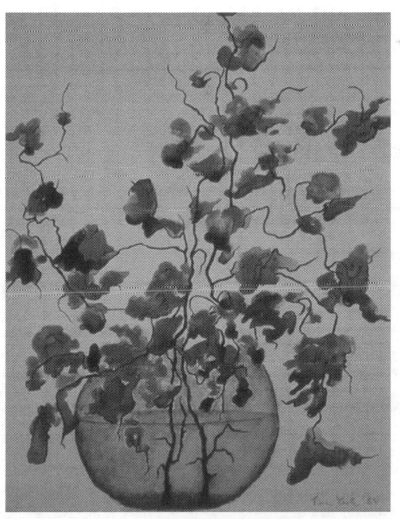

Bouganvilleas

INTRODUCTION

One of the main obstacles encountered in my development of the Neurophilosophy of Consciousness model of brain dynamics had consistently been to demonstrate the crucial role that the 'generative' human language faculty has in the generation of thoughts and an internal consciousness of 'self' as distinguished from the 'other' phenomenological perceptions in our external ongoing existential reality. I was logically forced to conclude that both language and thought are simultaneously cogenerated as 'bottoms up' information inputs to access higher cognitive levels in search of meanings. It implied the existence of an inherited generative grammar (proto-language) subject to constant modifications by phenomenological environmental circumstances (internal body proper and external environment). This is the classical stance of cognitive linguistics as opposed to psycholinguistics as elaborated below. This was expressed decades ago in Volume I of our model thus:

"Any comprehensive philosophy of natural languages, or meta-linguistics, must include considerations on syntax, semantics, referentials, phonology, truth values and pragmatics. Of these the most important and puzzling component remains semantics, a theory of meaning. We asked in a previous publication, what is it about certain marks, figures or a noise that endows them with such distinctive meanings? In our opinion, as we will expand on below, the most successful answers have identified in all of them 'propositional attitude' atomic particles which are neither language neutral nor analytically divorced from the reality it struggles to represent (see Quine famous book "Word and Object")." Consistent with our expressed underlying quotidian existential priorities, i.e., a biopsychosocial equilibrium (bps), we return back to this topic to argue again in favor of a hybrid synthesis of the unconscious, inherited generative neurolinguistic and the phenomenologically acquired psycholingustics. We hope this effort provides a justification for a 'team approach' in the management of mental illness.

ARGUMENTATION

In this brief analysis of human behavior in the decision-making process when confronted with either familiar or novel phenomenological circumstances in his biospheric niche, the human species is the center piece when trying to choose the best adaptive solution to this contingency. The source of the environmental challenge can be internal (body proper) or external, whether it arrives as a sensory perception input we can consistently/falsifiably measure or not. The latter is the case when the relevant input resists being framed into symbolic or sentential logic representation however predictable their consequences may turn out to be. How can we assign meaning to that relevant, consistent and predictable sensory or extrasensory input when we cannot use physical, real-world references to describe or explain its presence and the only option is to employ metaphysical logical structures to manage and resolve ambiguity and correctly choose the best individualized adaptive alternative where meanings are inferred from words and concepts (semantics) or from context (pragmatics)? When psycholinguists analyze the representation and function of language within the context of a physical human brain dynamics and neurolinguists take seriously the tenets of a real space-time mesoscopic reality requiring familiarity with the physical brain language acquisition, processing and discourse analysis in real time psychiatric wards, will they appreciate that both approaches incorporating the ontologically measured/observed and the epistemologically inferred Bayesian probabilities are simultaneously needed. The current metaphysical logic based cognitive linguistics with its esoteric cognitive grammar, conceptual metaphors and frame semantics need not look down to the physical brain embodied experiences of the real patient in the psycholinguist's office session. The 'form-function' correspondence stemming from symbolic/sentential logic leaves out the most important consideration criteria of 'truth content' forcing the theorists to resort to the conclusion of a mysterious functionalist 'emergence phenomena' of a general purpose or universal character belief ignoring the individualized ongoing circumstantial reality of the flesh and bones patient by interpreting language in terms of the universal concepts and seldom specific enough to a particularly environmentally acquired tongue, which must underlie its forms. A truth conditional theory of meaning is the un-articulated common denominator of ALL approaches, usually expressed as the 'coherence value' or the way a 'true sentence' relates to each other in a cognitive context. In so doing it is ignoring the more important empirical findings from the psychiatry/psychology practitioners. More important they ignore the individualized, unique and autonomous mental processes that underlie the acquisition, storage, production and understanding of speech and writing. The foregoing arguments should not be construed as an endorsement of an exclusive psycholinguistic practice approach but instead as a call for a joint team effort approach bringing both empirical and theoretical aspects of the problem to efficiently bear on the 'bps' equilibrium welfare of the real patient. Updating the diagnosing potential of mental illness by the cognitive linguistic approach is of the essence, as argued elsewhere, but ignoring the credible experiments of Broca and Wernicke establishing the modularity of language processing by proclaiming it is not separate from the rest of cognition, is a faith belief equivalent, just like declaring the irrelevance of a 'generative grammar' controlling linguistic communication is to the psycholinguist, an article of faith.

Having considered all historical arguments on 'meaning', whether 'referentialism' (words refer to things and their relationships in an actual or possible world) or Wittgenstein's 'use' (a conventionally assigned value within an existing social practice) and variations thereof, it has become clear that whatever theory of meaning we may want to elaborate, it can not be isolated from an obligatory co-evaluation of both 'syntax' (grammatical ordering of word relations to achieve maximum consistency for a given language) and 'pragmatics' (rules to achieve the maximum meaning content for a particular speech context). A truth-conditional theory of meaning is the un-articulated common denominator of all approaches, usually expressed as the 'coherence value' or the way a 'true sentence' relates to others in a cognitive context.

SUMMARY AND CONCLUSIONS

Cognitive linguist theorists have been consistent in denying autonomy to the brain based language faculty of the mind when they refuse to consider grammar in any other terms than its representational conceptualization; i.e., humans only learn languages by using them. In so doing they exclude the well established modularity of the human brain's structure and function as amply demonstrated by Broca, Wernicke and others. This means that language acquisition is neither unique nor autonomous, thereby ignoring self-evident neurosurgical observations to the contrary in support of the existence of a generative grammar. This way acquisition, storage and retrieval of language is not significantly different from the storage and retrieval of information from the rest of cognition. This leaves phonemes, morphemes, and syntax cognition as unrelated to the moderate Sapir-Whorf empirical world poetry model embedded in the experiences and interactivity of their users but exclusively in the conceptual domain of discourse.

As we have argued elsewhere, the phenomenological sensory perception (internal body proper and external environment) must precede the epistemological conceptualization. Humans conceptualize a given physical reality of interest/relevance whether measured, observed or deemed probable and not the other way around. Physical damage to Broca's human frontal neocortex causes language deficits whereas physical damage to left posterior, superior temporal gyrus results in Wernicke's language aphasia, both of which are correlated to mental aberrations.

Much later, during the decade of the fifties, theoretical linguistics, under the leadership of Noam Chomsky, incorporated scientific methodology into the philosophy of language effort and effectively did away with the Skinnerian behaviorist skepticism about the worth of the neurobiological approach to study the brain directly. In so doing, Chomsky opened a new search path to discover the meaning of mind and self-consciousness. However, Chomsky concentrated on the syntax aspect of language structure, describing how natural language practitioners are able to generate and select only well-formed strings of sentences in a recursive manner appropriate for that given language, without much effort on the part of the subject. The implied grammar selection thus generated during the syntactic parsing by the 'deep structures' in the brain is considered by us as the possible search for a best-fit semantic content in the generated sentences. Can't separate one from the other, is the meaning predicated on the syntax structure . . . . or vice verse? (Taken from "Neurophilosophy of Consciousness.", Volume I). The details of Fodor's Language of Thought (LOT) analysis is beyond the scope of this brief presentation.

Dr. Angell O. de la Sierra, Esq. Winter 2013 Deltona, Florida.
Ref.: http://delaSierra-Sheffer.net

End of Ch. 9

CHAPTER

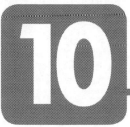

10 Controlling the Self Deceptive Syndrome

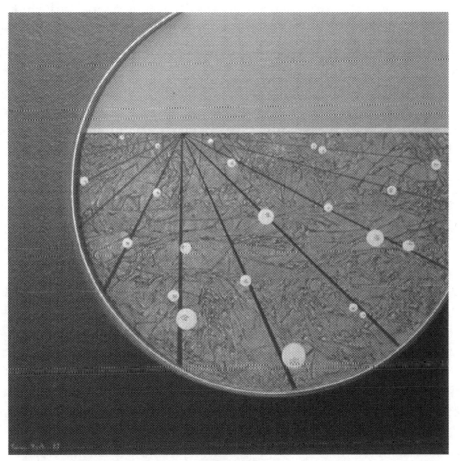

Cybernion

INTRODUCTION

In a nutshell, 'self deception' feelings during an ongoing decision-making process, had been a source of personal confusion for quite some time now thanks to modern scientific technology and mathematical logic sophistications. It is no longer as threatening even though it remains as enigmatic. We have abundantly analyzed elsewhere how the human brain consciously acquires and maintains a belief 'a' tailored to the individual's present and past existential circumstances while simultaneously being consciously aware of good evidence to the contrary in co-existing belief 'b'.

ARGUMENTATION

Belief 'a' responds to the exigent circumstances of sheer species survival imperatives shared with other subhuman species that subconsciously also act to stay alive, experience the neuro-hormone driven psychic state of emotional feelings while being assisted by the corresponding good feeling of being socially accepted to share a cooperative labor with others in the community. This we had coined as the adaptive biopsychosocial (bps) equilibrium strategy for species biological survival. In an evolving reality these beliefs are expected to be modified. How much? Belief 'a', which many, including Libet, et al, thought we had no conscious control of, has been shown by fMRI to be the result of a very conscious contrivance to survive, at all costs, and why not? Do we have choices? Yes we humans do. Here we part company with our beloved sub-humans sharing our vital chunk of biosphere turf and develop our belief 'b'.

Belief 'b' evolves in the direction and intensity that a given subjects' intellectual resources, experiences, interests, etc. permit. It is the meditative Sancho Panza of Don Quijote's meditations that exists in all of us, constantly warning and confusing us about dangers that maybe are there or not! Belief 'a' adaptively responds to existential phenomenological contingencies along biopsychosocial survival (BPS) guidelines, a problem solver. Belief 'b' reflects on the same contingency for effective solutions today AND the 'day after tomorrow'. Beyond the perceptual phenomenological input could there be additional, non-conventional sources of information input? Quare. We believe so and have elaborated on the conceptual mathematical logic evidence sustaining our model poem. It is fair to say that sometimes we wished we had less freely willed introspective access to plan 'a' or 'b' in response to ongoing, real space time contingencies. Poor Sancho Panza having to listen to himself and Don Quixote at the same time before deciding the next step! See "Meditaciones del Quijote".

I can only relate about how self-deception may represent a challenge if not an outright obstacle to self-knowledge and moral development. It is not easy to feel a stranger to yourself, consciously blind to your own moral failings while struggling to survive. Read on previous Volume V (Part II, YOGI) and you'll get to know about an embellished, fictional version of REAL experiences lived in flesh and blood.

When you meditate deep, like only a 'YOGI' can, you discover unexpected relations, not just the mathematical logic formulation best fitting your brain storm but the unconventional beauty in form and the dramatic simplification for the prepared analyst in search of the truths they hopefully contain. The Don Quijote in Sancho Panza's brain can do more than just battle fictional windmills, he can enjoy abstract beauty and reach transfinity while in search for . . . what?

Who can ignore 17th century Isaac Newton, who dare contrive a symbolic calculus representation to frame a credible explanation about the motions of the planets around the sun! Or the deceptively simple Pythagorean formulation $a^2 + b^2 = c^2$ that so brilliantly amalgamates geometry and numbers! See [5 Seriously Mind-Boggling Math Facts].

Need I mention Einstein 'alter ego' as captured in his formulas for special relativity, which embodies a whole new fancy way of looking at the cosmological multi-verse we conceptualize, an entirely new vision of a dynamical evolving phenomenological 'reality?' and our relationship to it. Suddenly reality is you and your brain capacity to explain it! To make a long story short I will give you what I consider the biggest simplification about the most complex conceptualization of the sensory experience that our 'alter ego' is capable of, under plan 'b'. Imagine Von Euler's alter ego genius representing the sensory sphere of our common experience as, e.g., a mathematical tetrahedron shape of four triangles, six edges (E) and four vertices (V) and faces (F). Applying pressure to its surface (F) will make it evolve into a sphere such that $V - E + F = 2$ will always be true of any other combination of faces, edges and vertices. Notice that any geometry, e.g., polygon, is a sphere in potency as it sequentially diminishes its size, as discussed above. This is a consistent but mind boggling fact that such a deceptively simple formulation explains so much about our metaphysical reality!. What reality is true? The ego existence or the superego dream if they both are consciously available? Are we one or the other? We submit 'a' and 'b' are both dynamically embedded into each other as a unit whole either one prevailing in control depending of the quality and nature of our inherited and acquired lifetime experiences.

What is puzzling is what determines the controlling influence in the conscious human choice of alternative (b), especially against survival self interest that fuels altruistic behaviors? What is the source of righteousness that guides Jesus sacrificial acts; Jesus of Nazarene, Mother Theresa of Calcutta, Mahatma Ghandi, Dalai Lama and other historical prophets? What is important IMHO, is the exemplary life they lived under adversity, when they had the conscious choice of a more comfortable alternative 'a'. The easiest explanation to justify this historical fact is to invoke the operation of a reciprocal information transfer process between a putative source in transfinity space time coordinates and a premotor neocortex. This represents the metaphysical logic equivalent of theosophical, agnostic, materialistic physical Gods. But, ultimately, within the context of an existential reality, brain dynamics model, it doesn't matter much for the vast majority of our species; if theosophical Gods do not exist, we will invent them if it helps to maintain ourselves inside the BPS norms of cooperative psychosocial conviviality.

This is an excerpt taken from the book "Neurophilosophy of Consciousness, Vol. V and YOGI." Published by Trafford, Inc. of Penguin Books.

EPILOGUE

This Vol. VI, Neurophilosophy of Consciousness may well be the last published account of my biopsychosocial (BPS) model of brain dynamics. Existential real time contingencies rightfully claim my priority attention. I hope that my controversial views on existential reality can be convincing and lead others in pursuing and improving on its content which we summarize as follows:

1) Existential, mesoscopic human functional reality is in the physical brain of the beholder. The ontological arguments constitute the most important element in the hybrid BPS synthesis.

2) Noumenal reality conceptualization is a goal for the creative mind to justify his conscious choice of model. The epistemological arguments constitute a necessary but insufficient element in the Epistemontological hybrid.

3) That goal is to explain how may the classic, continuous macro aggregates of unit dimensional quantized, discrete, micro physical particles be fundamentally different from the same quantum particle it originated from? What is the justification for having two seemingly paradoxical but consciously willed views on the same fundamental reality? One view describes the quotidian, entropic, spontaneous functional reality of preserving the species integrity from extinction by subconscious deployment of adaptive BPS survival strategies to counter real or probable, familiar or novel dangerous contingencies as they enter our human vital 4-d sp ace time coordinates. The opposing view, of lower priority in deployment for most humans, while analogous in deployment, seems oriented to maintain the same adaptive biopsychosocial equilibrium with the evolving environment in guarantee of the human species survival across generations, notwithstanding our species inferior adaptive resources compared to other subhuman species. The justification for this human centered evolution of complexity is explained better by Bergson's "Creative Evolution" into the uncertain future. One may ask, why bother, why not let the better adapted species take over as Darwinian style 'survival of the fittest' evolution successfully predicts? What makes humans survive across generations while better fit subhuman species become recorded history? As a limited species humans can describe or explain the 'how' it happens; the 'why' becomes the challenge to reach and conjecture/speculate to satiate that burning curiosity psychosis of some humans. Why humans? What about them makes them the 'chosen' ones? Chosen by who, what, when, where, why?? At first sight, the answer is simplistic, because humans are the ones describing, explaining or speculating in language narratives when their physical brains are healthy, experience psychic emotions of happiness especially when their narratives are shared with other social members of his biological 'pack' working. We will never know if any evolved, advanced subhuman species is doing the same in their apparently primitive language and some future day will develop unsuspected technologies, egalitarian constitutions, marvelous engineering masterpieces and expressive works of art. Until such 'paradise' emerges and from a functional point of view, we are talking about a neo Copernican

revolution with the human species, for good or for bad, at the center of the universe s(he) measures or invents and narrates in the form of model poems for self indulgence or self sacrifice in behalf of others, as the case may be!

Thus, in the functional domain we experience emotions of opposite valence and we witness altruistic behavior against self interest. Consequently, an innate curiosity about our origins and destiny after death naturally takes hold of your thoughts. Within the unconscious framework of life preservation we wonder about the living and what functionally seems like non-living to sensory experience. Some are e.g., able to consistently measure energy transfer when living green leaves are exposed to light sources, then they see mitochondria and test for chlorophyll inside the plant cells. A quantum of discrete particulate matter seems to control the macro observation of the resulting energy transfer. The resulting explanatory quantum model contains phenomenological functional measurements and metaphysical logic concepts, both sharing a side of the same coin trying to explain the 'how' by reconciling the functional phenomenological with the non-physical poem. If the functional aggregates of particulate discrete particles are derived from the original unit mass particle one needs to explain why the need for different metrics? The explanation for the 'why' is even more complex. The innate curiosity for the source of consistent but ineffable feelings or qualia fuels the restless imagination into the creation of transcendental belief models that again harmonizes within the tenets on the historical benefits of adopting an adaptive BPS equilibrium strategy. The same scenario holds for the search for explanations of 'life'. What animates physical particles into self sustaining motion? What animates nucleoprotein crystals from Rous Sarcoma virus into living invasive activity. Can robots become animated? Can we synthesize life in the laboratory at will? All of the questions have one thing in common, the functionally inert matter did not spontaneously come into an organized living state un-assisted, in all cases the 'living state' required mediation of a living organism to 'assist' in the transformation. Where does life come from? We still need credible, reliable and coherent answers. If we cannot discover the answer, we will invent one with predictable powers while we continue the search for the ultimate causality, slowly but without a pause. Penrose-Hameroff microtubular receptor proteins ubiquity in membrane channels poem is as convincing as the spontaneous self sustaining, self causation emergence of negentropic order magic or the central role dark baryonic reciprocal information transfer DNA/RNA receptors requiring that super symmetry environmental stability that propitiates the trans-generational biological survival of Homo Sapiens. To follow are the mathematical logic justifications for the epistemological component of our BPS model of brain dynamics.

End of Ch. 10

Dirac's <bra-ket> Vector Analysis Update

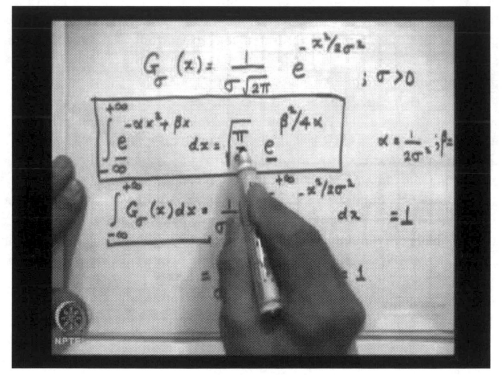

Dirac's Delta Function

INTRODUCTION

Anyone who has ever stood up in front of a classroom to address his/her students will tell you that simplicity is a worthwhile pragmatic and a theoretical virtue goal iff the expected and appropriate pedagogic results are aimed at the student and not the teacher, independent of the corresponding level of complexity to be communicated. There is a presumption that 'selling/ marketing' an idea by a professor implies there must be a 'buyer' student for a pedagogical transaction to be completed. Unless, of course, the professor, consciously knowing (or not) is engaged in a self-serving soliloquy phrased as primitive, 'self-evident' propositions and often expressed as either theology or probable/statistical science inspired radical extremist pronouncements. Yet, a complex and changing nature, in its dynamic evolutionary progression in our 4-d space time existential reality, opts to reveal its complexity to human narrators in the form of the simplest possible model-poems solution that are compatible with the narrators' brain dynamics' phenomenology and combinatorial limitations, as amply detailed in our other publications. We now expand on the justifications for our general poem on the evolution of complexity as discussed under "The Immanent Invariant and the Transcendental Transforming Horizons." See Ch. 12, "Nurophilosophy of Consciousness.", Vol. IV and Vol. V.

ARGUMENTATION

If we ever have expectations from our biopsychosocial (BPS) model poem of human brain dynamics ever evolving into a reliable theory of everything (TOE) it must satisfy some minimum requirements as detailed below. The most important requirement being that the model's principles must be rationally/logically justified as a general/universal application to any aspect of human enquiry, whether its content is exclusively epistemological idealism or an exclusively pragmatic, methodological and empirical type. The model approach can also take the form of a hybrid combination of idealism and empiricism in nature like our own Epistemontological hybrid tracking this super-complex reality as it evolves in our 4-d space-time biosphere niche. We hope that our consciously free willed choice of simplified analytic mathematical elaboration is readable and reaches the curiosity of all informed readers in any discipline. In the search for an adequate universal mathematical formulation we had to justify the need for 'a priori' metaphysical elements (including philosophy, theosophy, mathematics, etc.) and the need for 'a posteriori' pragmatic/physical elements as emerging from scientific methodology measurements/observations of nature. It is due time to rationally integrate pragmatic empiricism and rational idealism as a functional unit whole in living human reality as justified by consistent, falsifiable and predictable results from quantum theory based probability theory and/or Bayesian statistics including theosophically-justified speculations and conjectures as exemplified by the famous Leibniz Monadology or our own sub-model arguments for the probability of a reciprocal information transfer between the human pre-motor neo-cortex attractor phase space and unspecific space-time n-1 coordinates in transfinity as mediated by the human brain baryonic dark matter DNA/RNA receptor site.

Our central focus on the human biopsychosocial (BPS) existential reality equilibrium adapting our species to familiar (or new) contingencies presenting a potential threat to human survival has led us to seriously consider how may the human inferior adaptive limitations to a changing environmental landscape (compared to other evolved subhuman species) notwithstanding, the human species have survived across generations performing the wondrous evolutionary technological and societal transformations other species are innately incapable of? What keeps the human species at the helm of the Bergsonian evolution of complexity, above the mere BPS survival other evolved subhuman species share? Intuitively, the easy answer is to search for entities outside/beyond our immediate 4-d space-time earth biosphere environment that specifically/selectively influence the human species. The same intuition, always looking for simplicity, makes you posit the probability that **before** being the architect responsible for the wondrous transformation the human species has **first** to be alive, healthy and psychosocially adapted, in equilibrium with his immediate, individualized environment. It makes intuitive sense to suspect that such transfinite source should **first** be able to functionally equip humans with the resources to offset the inferior adaptive capabilities in the biosphere milieu and **second** 'create' the super symmetry transfinite conditions that minimizes the probability of disruptive transfinite radiation affecting our biosphere. Part of that radiation may exclusively reach the human premotor neocortex to anticipate damaging radiation events.

The careful reader may have noticed the posited existence of two unreachable infinities at play, the micro sub-Planckian manifold actively controlling the local events and the cosmological manifold controlling transfinity. We immediately wonder what resources may our poorly adapted human species to life on earth, with its known phenomenal and brain combinatorial limitations, may mobilize to stay alive and become the architect of this wondrous civilization?? Can anyone imagine better adapted subhuman species like Rhesus monkeys or ants, roaches, etc creating optogenetic and gene transplant technology controlling DNA/RNA transduction, the same way transfinite radiation does? How else may any human being explain, if not describe, the cosmological order being influenced by natural complex asymmetries evolving to become the super symmetries that minimize universal damaging radiation impacting the earth and facilitating the reciprocal information transfer mechanism between humans and transfinity sources. We need a model poem formula that operates both at the local mesoscopic biosphere and at the cosmological order level that is compatible with the structural/functional idiosyncrasies of a human brain.

We have climbed on the shoulders of Dirac and others to formulate probable approximations compatible with all disciplines created by the same human physical brain. What follows is a brief summary of the salient technical features still undergoing revisions with the joint 'help' of the good willed informed literati and the ill willed vicious trollers that plague some HiQ online listings. ☺

For details on these formulations see Blog site: http://angelldls.wordpress.com/; <http://angelldls.wordpress.com/author/angelldls/> and http://delaSierra-Sheffer.net For the present needs of this brief article on the merits of a modified Dirac notation we only highlite the possible interactive correlations between the local and transfinite sources of information and the need for functional approximations requiring a minimization of relevant interacting variables at both extremes of the the spectrum, the phenomenologically invisible levels of activity at both the subplanckian local level and the cosmological level. At the micro level our sub model requires the attainment of supersymmetry to posit the presence of monopoles and gravitons to facilitate the influence of low intensity transfinite radiation on the local genetic transduction process of the brain neuron target cell via dark matter baryon receptor. The ongoing debate centers on **what** sub atomic micro particle is involved in the information transfer, the neutrino, the axion, etc. and **where** does it originate? We concentrate on the measurable **how** and understress the theosophical **why.**

The charge free 'neutrino' is the candidate of choice to penetrate un-opposed miles deep geological barriers to reach the buried instrument receptors at CERN. Radioactive, stable hydrogen H_1 (spin1) atoms are known to spontaneously emit ½ spin electrons during their Beta decay process to a suitable acceptor of opposite-1/2 spin leaving the originally stable spin 1 source spin—½ deficient as measured. In our model this naturally decaying or radiation-induced hydrogen atom can be on either side of the reciprocal communication path, the human brain cell or a transfinity source of radiation. It is assumed that path direction is a function of need to insure the availability of an BPS survival adaptive response to challenging environmental contingencies. All experiments confirm the same fractional deficit attending radioactive degradation. If, as the result of nucleosynthesis activity immediately after the Big Bang, dark baryonic particle radiation found its way into cellular DNA/RNA is not as farfetched as it seems to arm chair idealist theorists who rather prefer the charming argument of the 'massless' physical particle http://en.wikipedia.org/wiki/Weyl_equation! ☺ To justify the deep penetration of the particulate matter it has to be charge neutral and only microgravitational forces in the form of magnetic monopoles will do to avoid the dipolar nature of electromagnetic induced fields. Enter gravitons and Dirac who questioned what good theoretical reason explains why the un-observed/undetected monopoles could not exist within a quantum theory framework? It made more overall sense to posit its existence than its absence. It is clear that a consistent, falsifiable observation or a physics-laboratory experiment should not necessarily be always considered as a check on the necessary and sufficient proof of its truth content or even the conceptual mathematical correctness of the symbolic or sentential representations of the current Dirac-equation solution. When both the physical empirical measurement of a real effect and a metaphysical logic are hybridized, the confirmation of the electron particle physical mass, graviton or monopoles structure become a goal whose detection ability in the electron physics lab is still beyond reach, if ever.

The best way to describe the temporal evolution of the multidimensional complexity of any quantum state in a linear scalar progression (like the way our brain linearizes sensory information input) is to update the Schrodinger and Hamiltonian space into a Hilbert space that may take into account any vector ray projection path direction. This allows for the differential representation of a multiple number of relevant variable paths interacting between themselves as one single resultant package. Each of the participating quantum states can be represented in the standard Bracket notation where $\langle \phi | \psi \rangle$, consisting of a left part, $\langle \phi |$, called the bra and a right part, $| \psi \rangle$, called the ket. The notation was invented by Paul Dirac. The effective use requires minimizing the number of relevant dependent variants by approximations as they affect the phenomenological perceptualization of an independent invariant unit dimensional physical particle or aggregations thereof. In a TOE model any conserved value, matter, momentum, etc. will do. It should be remembered that the progression range of all of the N particles (positive integer > 0) individual 3-d x, y, z dependent variables inputs as they project into a Hilbert space of 6N real dimensions gets reduced to a single valued function output. Quantum theory integrates the 3-d configuration space plus the 6-d Hilbert space into a 9-d space replacing the classical brain phase space. Each projective ray path represents a frame-independent Schrodinger wave function where the operator defines the appropriate frame of reference. If one path harmonic ray rotates stretches, etc., they all do (at right angles to each other or orthogonal) except when several points co-habit and interact in same 2-d plane (not the line axis!) where each point coordinates lies (each eigen value—momentum, position, spin—etc.—defining its probability amplitude) have conflicting physical existence. Not all possible observables can be simultaneously measured, eg., position and spin of particle, giving rise to Heisenberg' uncertainty principle. At the sub-planckian scale (10-33 cm) quantum gravity space is a lattice and we can have an infinity of dimensions for an open ended forever-expanding universe. Each of these mutually perpendicular basic rays represents a particular potential behavior of a quantum system and the set of all basic rays for a given property constitute the relativistic frame of reference in Hilbert space. Orthogonality provides for potential activities that are classically distinct or mutually exclusive. Also, the number of dimensions needed in this abstract space corresponds to the number of choices available for the quantum system, and this, as we have just seen, can go to infinity. In such cases the product of their Hilbert spaces gives rise to the "entangled states" of the Einstein-Podolsky-Rosen (EPR) effect. In Hilbert space the ubiquitous electron can be in all possible places all the time. In this respect a Hilbert space concept is more than adequate to carry on the baton for the representation of the quotidian familiar everyday world.

In general terms the Dirac notation below satisfies the identities inside the brackets < > where $\tilde{\psi}$ is the complex conjugate. By mathematical logic transformations the general terms can be further transformed into operational functional representations allowing a 'visualization' of the temporal course of evolution of any unit dimensional invariant particle aggregates as they project their evolutionary progression into the multidimensional Hilbert space allowing for predictable warnings about probable future happenings in our biosphere of interest.

$$\langle \phi | \tilde{O} | \psi \rangle \equiv \langle \phi | \tilde{O} \psi \rangle$$

$$\langle \phi | \psi \rangle \equiv \int_{-\infty}^{\infty} \bar{\phi} \psi \, dx,$$

SUMMARY AND CONCLUSIONS

If the objective reader still considers recorded history as at least a reliable guide as to how complexity has evolved from memorable Aristotelian times to our convulsive 21th. Century, it should be obvious that each historical period had the task to reconcile the immanent/pragmatic, phenomenological 'seen' and the transcendental, relevant epistemological 'unseen'. We can summarily mention Aristotle's analytical guide in his 'ceteris paribus' strategy to minimize the number of postulates or hypotheses to make your model poem more credible. Even St. Thomas Aquinos recognized in the Middle Ages how natural laws of simplicity adequately guide the course of universal evolution. Likewise Kant—in the *Critique of Pure Reason*—supports the idea of minimizing the number of non-phenomenological assumptions/principles contained in 'Pure Reason'-based arguments underlying scientists' theorizing about nature. If true and sufficient, as consistently verified by all human observers, whether philosophers, experimentalists, and/or practitioners, why muddle the truth content goal with the claim of exclusivity based on pronouncements about subjective radical sensory or extrasensory individualized experiences. Why not heed today the pragmatic, universal suggestions from 14th. Century Occam's Razor, Galileo or Newton's *Principia Mathematica?* Why settle for the self serving pomp and circumstance of superfluous causalities as defended by the radicalized arm chair physicalist theorists or the experimentalists, practitioners and philosophers? On the other radical extreme, why should anyone accept as the exclusive truth the metaphysical, subjective, individualized content of a physical human brain's theosophy-inspired cosmogony experiences? Three centuries ago the chemist Lavoisier ridiculed the hypothetical metaphysical 'phlogiston' as the exclusive explanation of phenomenological chemical reactions observed, a rejection based exclusively on mathematical logic principles that minimizes the arbitrariness of non phenomenal brainstorms. Again, mesoscopic existential reality demands the easiest and simplest explanations to explain the realities a healthy physical human brain experiences. To guaranty the maximum probability of truth content we need to integrate the maximum number of empirical consistent, falsifiable human measurements/ observations resting on logical deductions and a bare minimum of axiomatic-based model poems. This is true of all disciplines created and narrated by the exclusive, individualized human brain dynamic activity whether we like it or not. The polarization we witness between the hands-on physical ontologists and the arm chair metaphysical epistemologists in current 21st. century debate on 'consciousness' seem to rely exclusively on the burden of proof summoned in defense of one's point of view, thanks to the magic experimental results coming from modern technology, especially when they score high in the predictive value. All things being hopefully considered, the undersigned author still believes that providing credible arguments rooted on solid consistent measured/observed empirical facts refuting competing theories is more important as a starting point in the debate as to the probable truth content of our conscious model choice. A case in point is the un-necessary **causality** debate on probable truth content between the undeniable linguistic elegance of arm chair mathematic theorists and the hands-on cold probable/statistical laboratory facts reports of real time-space practitioners. Considering the evolving super complexity of both the physical human brain structure/function and that of the universe how dare either extreme version proclaim the exclusivity of their domain of discourse at the exclusion of the rival unknown other? Why do materialist physicists knowingly posit the existence of two coexisting but different ontologies in the mind-brain dualist interpretation of the human brain dynamics when they should know that etymologically ontology belongs to the phenomenological domain whereas mind is an epistemological denotation? Why not share and learn from each other including the justifiable arguments of each other in a current but evolving hybrid Epistemontological synthesis as we have proposed and have exhaustingly analyzed in our BPS model of brain **dynamics.

The reason we briefly discussed the Dirac methodology is because we also believe that if our model aspirations of becoming an universal theory of everything (TOE) we should justify the BPS model poem of brain dynamics as applicable to any area of human enquiry regardless of being formulated as an epistemology or methodology principle. Because we consider both principles as two coexisting, inseparable aspects of the same mesoscopic existential reality in our human species biosphere.

Dr. Angell O. de la Sierra, Esq.
Deltona, Florida Spring, 2013-04-27.